Esophageal Cancer

Real-Life Stories
from Patients and Families

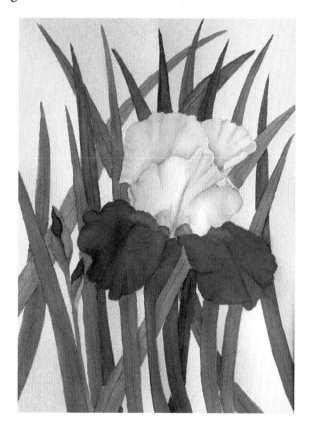

Edited by

Ellen R. Abramson

Red/White Iris
Cover and title page artwork by Vincent Maiorana
Reprinted with permission

Cover design by Aki Yao
Learning Design & Publishing
Medical School Information Services

Published by Michigan Publishing
University of Michigan Library

ISBN: 978-1-60785-357-2

DEDICATION

With heartfelt thanks to Dr. Mark Orringer whose care, leadership and innovations have meant so much to so many.

INTRODUCTION

"The same way, every day" is a mantra heard frequently in the operating rooms and patient wards at our hospital as a reminder by my mentor and colleague, Mark Orringer, MD, about the importance of being vigilant and attentive to the care of our patients, particularly those who have undergone an esophagectomy. Esophageal cancer is a devastating diagnosis for which patients often need chemotherapy, radiation as well as surgical treatment. During an esophagectomy, removing the cancer requires removal of the majority of the esophagus, the fibromuscular tube through which food passes before entering the stomach. In order to restore swallowing, the stomach is reconfigured into a tube that is repositioned through the chest and sutured to the remaining esophagus.

Each story in this collection describes the courage and strength that these patients and their families exhibit following an esophagectomy when a patient must learn to adapt to changes in his or her ability to eat, to handle side effects such as nausea, abdominal pain, regurgitation and dumping syndrome.

As you read these stories, please consider that these individuals have endured considerable physical pain and emotional anguish. At the time of diagnosis, patients might experience disbelief and shock. After a sometimes-bewildering array of testing and consultation, after completing treatment and getting through their operation, patients may have numerous questions: Will the cancer return? Will further treatment be needed? How will I be able to eat? Such questions and many more reflect the potential loss of control and loss of independence that we all might experience in similar situations.

In 2002, Lori Flint, RN, started our esophagectomy support group to provide a venue where our patients and their families could work through these questions with others who have had to address similar concerns. As families, friends and even strangers provide their care and support, patients begin a remarkable transformation into recovery. We are indebted to these men and women and their families for sharing their life stories.

Andrew C. Chang, M.D.
John Alexander Distinguished Professor of Thoracic Surgery
Associate Professor of Surgery and Section Head
University of Michigan Medical School

PREFACE

For the past eleven years, I have worked as a fundraiser for the University of Michigan Health System. Before that, I worked as a fundraiser for the American Red Cross, and earlier yet for the Ross School of Business at the University of Michigan. In all, I have been a development officer for twenty years. To many people, the idea of asking for money is terrifying. They are afraid of doing it wrong, embarrassing themselves, being perceived as rude or inappropriate. And they are afraid of rejection. I, too, have felt all those fears.

I have learned, and I encourage colleagues and friends who would like to be able to ask for support to remember, that we are not asking for ourselves. We are not even asking for the University of Michigan Health System or the other organizations we serve. We are asking on behalf of the people who will benefit from the support. I am asking on behalf of the patients and families who will benefit from the medical research that philanthropy makes possible. I am asking on behalf of the patients who will be cared for by doctors who received scholarships or whose education was enriched through private support.

When I began fundraising for U-M Thoracic Surgery, I began to hear stories – stories of esophageal cancer patients who survived, stories of husbands and wives whose spouses had passed away but who were grateful for the extra several months or several years which their care at U-M Thoracic Surgery had made possible. I realized that these patients and families – and people like them – were the people for whom I was asking for support.

I became aware of the Esophagectomy Support Group and was warmly welcomed by the group and given the opportunity to attend several meetings. I shared with them the idea of this book – a compilation of stories of patients who had undergone esophagectomy surgery. I offered two purposes for the creation of this book. One was the opportunity to have an additional helpful resource for esophageal cancer patients, and their families, who were facing this surgery. The other was the opportunity to dedicate this book to Dr. Mark Orringer, the surgeon for many of these patients, and someone to whom they are all so deeply grateful.

It is a great privilege to help people make a meaningful difference in the lives of others, in a way that is also deeply meaningful to them. That's the way I look at my fundraising, and that's the way I look at this book. I hope that there will be many people for whom this book is deeply meaningful.

Ellen R. Abramson
Associate Director of Development
University of Michigan Health System

If you are interested in knowing how you can help advance research on esophageal cancer and other thoracic cancers and conditions, please contact the University of Michigan Health System Office of Medical Development at (734) 998-7705.

CONTENTS

Dedication

Introduction

Preface

Acknowledgments

1. *Why The Esophagectomy Support Group Is So Important To Me,....*   1
    by Lori Flint

2. *In Sickness and In Health*, by Andy A.............................   5

3. *The New Normal*, by Anne A.   9

4. *Know That Life Is A Gift*, by Clare L.   13

5. *Tales From The Blindside*, by Connie L.   19

6. *My Path To Surviving and Thriving*, by John K....................   37

7. *Each New Day Is A Blessing*, by Ken S...........................   43

8. *My Esophagectomy Story*, by Paul E..............................   55

9. *My Toughest Marathon*, by Peter H..............................   61

10. *Surviving Esophageal Cancer*, by Russ P.........................   67

11. *My Journey: Esophageal Cancer to Transhiatal Esophagectomy,* 71
 ("THE"), by Stephen P.

12. *Esophagectomy Story,* by Vincent M.................................. 77

13. *My Experience With The Esophagectomy Support Group,*.............. 85
 by Tiffany Staal

 Biography of Mark Orringer, M.D............................... 89

 Resources.. 91

 About the Editor.. 93

ACKNOWLEDGMENTS

Thank you to Dr. Andrew Chang, the John Alexander Distinguished Professor of Thoracic Surgery, and Head of Thoracic Surgery at the University of Michigan, for his support and partnership on this project.

I am very grateful to Lori Flint, RN, and Tiffany Staal, RN, for their enthusiasm for this book idea, and their kindness in reaching out to members of the Esophagectomy Support Group.

A special thank you goes to Jasna Markovac, Senior Director, Learning Design and Publishing, Medical School Information Services at the University of Michigan. It was Jasna who suggested the idea for this book when I shared with her about the remarkable courage of our esophagectomy patients and their families in the face of tremendous challenge. I am grateful for Jasna connecting me with her colleague Karen Kost, Associate Publisher. Karen provided the step-by-step guidance and support that transformed a series of stories into a book. I have enjoyed the process of creating this book, and know that it would not have happened without the services provided by Jasna, Karen, and MSIS Learning Design and Publishing.

Finally, my most profound thanks go to the authors whose stories appear in this book. I am deeply grateful for their courage in writing these stories and their generosity in sharing them.

Ellen R. Abramson

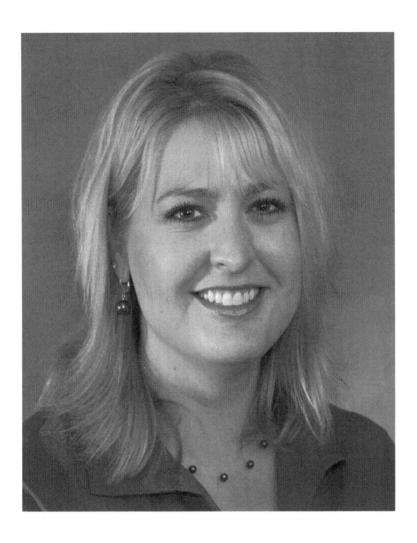

Lori Flint, RN

Chapter 1

Why The Esophagectomy Support Group Is So Important To Me

by Lori Flint, RN,
Thoracic Surgery Nurse 1997-2013

The support group has not only changed my nursing career, but the way I look at my personal life. I have learned so much from all of the folks who have gone through the meetings, sharing their stories, their initial struggles, and learning that having a good attitude, family/friend support, and staying busy will help you get through anything!

In the beginning

The support group came about sometime in 2002, although I really cannot remember the exact date. It started, by getting daily calls from the same patient. He was trying to get adjusted to his new way of life after surgery. The calls ranged from, 'What was he supposed to eat?, Why was he not hungry?, What was his wife supposed to do with him?'. He would periodically talk about his prior history as an alcoholic and the support he got from Alcoholics Anonymous. He kept talking about how he felt a support group would help him during his recovery from surgery. Finally, after a few weeks of daily calls (and those also calling with similar issues), I told him that - if he would help me - we could see about starting a support group. With the help and support of Dr. Orringer, and the thoracic surgery staff - including Sharon Fox, RN - the esophagectomy support group was started. I never thought it would grow the way it has, but am very proud of where it is today.

The first several meetings were small and we had a hard time finding a room that would work for all to find and feel comfortable during the discussion. As we continued to work on this, we were able to engage a very special patient, who was many years out from his esophagectomy. (He still comes to offer his advice on living with his 'new plumbing'.) He was on his way to Florida, when he came to that meeting. The patient who was the reason I got this support group started told me that talking with this patient helped him to turn the corner, and made a huge difference in his life and his overall wellbeing. It actually all had to do with eating strawberries. He was told if eating strawberries affected him when he ate them, then he should not eat the strawberries! This is when I knew we had to keep the support group going. Even if we helped just this one person, then it was all worth it. Little did I realize, not only would it help so many, but it also helped me be a better nurse to those going through this ordeal, from initial diagnosis to dealing with the life changes after their esophagectomy.

Through the years

We continued to try to change, improve and get the word out about the support group to help as many as we could. We started with a list of patients that others could email, and posted this on our website. As a suggestion from a family member, we were able to video one of our meetings for others to view if they could not make the support group here in Ann Arbor. This was actually funded by a patient's family; the patient had lost his battle with esophageal cancer. It was a great gift, that allowed many a chance to see how all the patients looked following surgery, as well as listen to what their initial struggles were and what they did about them and how they are today.

We would get calls from all across the country, as there are very few esophagectomy support groups. These folks would ask about the group and ask the patients on the email list all kinds of questions. I believe the patients, as they went through the meetings and answered their emails, realized how important their input was and how much they were helping others. That is an amazing feeling.

Changing of the guard

When I was looking to change my nursing role the hardest part was trying to figure out what would happen to the support group. It was a part of me, a part of 'my family', and I wanted to make sure I could continue it until it could be supported by another nurse. With knowing I could do that, I did change my nursing role. Of course, I was also able to 'support' the support group, until Tiffany came on board. Then I felt 'my family' was well cared for even though I was no longer there ☺.

Tincture of time

I wanted to make sure to point something out as you read this, whether you have just started the journey with esophageal disease or esophageal cancer, are looking at having the surgery, or have had the surgery. Know that it may not always turn out the way it was planned; remember to take it one day at a time and try to stay as positive as you can. You will be able to eat again, but this 'New Normal' will not be the same as now; it may be smaller food amounts, not right before bed, or not certain kinds of food.

I hope that if you are able to get to even one support group to see folks that have had the surgery and listen to how they have recovered, as well as read these stories, and see the video, it will help you make the best decision for you, and your disease process (which can be different for each person).

If surgery is set for you or done, and you are working to make it through the initial recovery period, know that you are not alone. Although each person is their own individual with different symptoms, there are many common threads and you can use all that you learn to help guide your steps to make it easier, one day at a time. Sharon Fox, one of the first thoracic surgery nurses, used to say the hardest pill to take is the 'tincture of time'. Just remember it will take time - along with support - and a positive attitude.

My gratitude

I want to make sure I thank Dr. Mark Orringer. I feel very fortunate and am a better nurse and person having had the honor to work alongside him all those many years. It was truly a privilege and I am forever grateful to him.

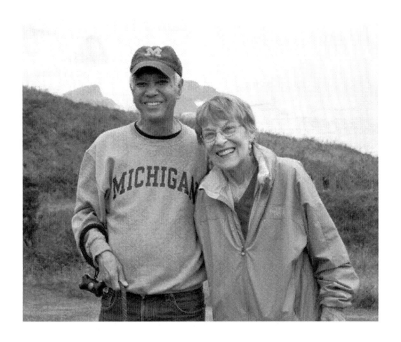

Andy and Anne A.

Chapter 2

In Sickness And In Health

by Andy A.,
Husband/Caregiver

Most of the spring and early summer of 2008, my wife, Anne, was having 'stomach' indigestion pains for which she started taking Tums. That did not seem to do the trick, so our family physician suggested a prescription medication. A month later at another appointment, Anne continued to complain. So, our family physician ordered a 'scope' of her stomach for September 2008. (A side note: Anne joined me in retirement in June 2008, and then this happened.)

I remember that day like it was yesterday. It is NEVER a good sign that when you are in post-procedure recovery and the doctor who performed the procedure pulls the curtain and looks for a chair. As he pulled the pictures up on the computer, he said something about the darker areas. All I can remember him saying is, "Until we get the test results back, I will not know for sure. However, I do this procedure every day, and I think it is cancer in the esophagus." From that moment, both Anne and I were in shock, in a haze, and very, very scared. I am not even sure what the checkout lady said.

However - and this is not an exaggeration - by the time we walked into our house (we live here in Ann Arbor) we received a phone call from our family physician. She said, "This is the worst possible news. This is what you are now going to do." And she listed who she was getting for the oncologist and radiologist and that we would hear back very soon.

Unlike others we know that have received similar bad news, we did not go to the internet to learn all we could about esophageal cancer. It just sounded too scary and we did not know any more than our family physician was on top of it and that the University of Michigan Medical Center was world class. We were, 'In good - the best –

5

hands'. We did not even know about the existence of the Esophageal Cancer Support Group right in our own back yard.

Over the course of the next two months, Anne received her radiation and chemotherapy, and we met Lori Flint and Dr. Mark Orringer, who monitored Anne's progress to surgery. Surgery had to be re-scheduled a couple of times because the radiation and chemo therapies took their toll and Anne needed more time to get her strength back. Surgery was finally done on April 2, 2009. She was in the hospital about twice as long as expected because of other, non-related surgery issues. I remained by her side 24/7 in the hospital, only coming home for a quick shower.

Recovery was slow but steady. Unlike most of the other patients, Anne had difficulty swallowing and had to see Dr. Orringer three times to be dilated. It was not easy watching Dr. Orringer put this seemingly large hose down my wife's throat as she gagged. At the third visit, Dr. Orringer said that he would watch me do the dilation because I would be the one to do it from now on at home. "Are you kidding me?" I said to myself. "I can hardly watch him do it - how in the world was I going to dilate my wife at home?"

But when you love someone and you work together, with each dilation it became easier for me to do and, I think, easier for Anne. For the first year or so, we dilated fairly frequently - perhaps every two to three weeks. It has become so infrequent now, I can't remember the last time we dilated. And, we are down to the optional annual visit with her oncologist, Dr. Susan Urba. This April 1, 2015 is her six-year anniversary, and we thank God for this blessing.

The Esophageal Cancer Support Group is excellent for pre-surgery information and post-surgery support. Looking back, I still feel that if we had known about the Group, we would not have attended pre-surgery meetings because of our fear of knowing more then we wanted to know. We fully embrace the value of the Group and have attended many meetings these past five years. We all benefit from everyone's stories, experiences, outcomes, and suggestions for dealing with the 'New Normal', as Lori would say.

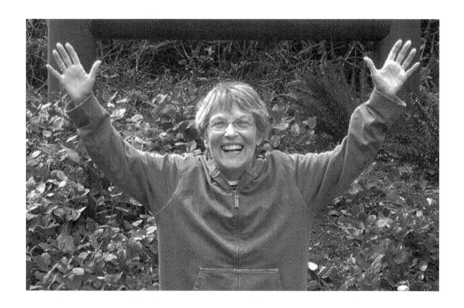

Anne A., at 14 ½ months after surgery

Chapter 3

The New Normal

by Anne A.

I was so looking forward in June 2008 when I retired to join my husband, who had been retired since 2005. However, after my annual physical in July, my primary family doctor suggested that I have an endoscopy to check out my chronic heartburn complaints. Everything changed in September when the doctor who performed the endoscopy told us (my husband was there) that I had Stage I esophageal cancer. I was in shock and may not have heard anything else.

By the time we got home, our primary family doctor was on the phone saying she just got the news, and here is the plan we must follow and who she was going to try to get for our oncologist, radiologist and surgeon. We just listened and over the next few months followed the plan, somewhat in a daze. Unlike some people, we were afraid to know more about this cancer by looking it up on the internet. We did not know about the Esophageal Cancer Support Group.

We met Dr. Orringer prior to the surgery, and he explained everything and drew his famous sketch on the exam table's paper of what the surgery was going to accomplish. We still have that drawing, and I still can hear him say, "I am going to do my part and I will do it right. Now you must do your part and walk three miles per day." My surgery was done by Dr. Orringer on April 2, 2009. My family tells me that after the surgery, Dr. Orringer was very pleased with the outcome and how I did during the six-hour surgery. My stay in the hospital was a little longer than the ten-day average. I was in for twenty-one days because of unrelated existing conditions with my lungs.

I am now four and a half years out and feel very blessed that I had the best team of doctors here at the University of Michigan Medical

Center. It has been a slow but steady recovery, and the beginning of my *New Normal*. First of all, unlike most patients, I have had to dilate myself (actually Dr. Orringer trained my husband to do the dilation). At first we were doing it a couple of times a week but started to decrease the frequency as time went along. Today, we may dilate once every six to eight weeks 'just to keep in practice', or when I feel it would help my eating.

Like most of the other patients, I must sleep on a slightly inclined bed (two inch bricks at the head of the bed) with a wedge-pillow and I cannot eat very large meals. I frequently snack between meals. If I eat something within two hours of going to bed at night, I may have a reaction. So far I have had two bile episodes, which were awful.

If I want to exercise or go anywhere, I do it before I eat because it is difficult for me to walk right after I have eaten. I am a small person and I know there is just a limited amount of space in my chest cavity for my heart, lungs and now my stomach. It is almost comical to see us check into a motel when traveling; the luggage cart is more than half full of two large black trash bags that contain my pillows.

This is my *New Normal*. It took some getting used to, but with time I have accepted it and have adjusted to it. Life is GOOD. I am indebted to my surgeon Dr. Orringer, my oncologist Dr. Susan Urba and my radiologist Dr. Hyman and the rest of my medical team. A special mention must be made of Lori Flint who guided me through the surgery process with calls, setting appointments, and encouragement. And a special thanks to her for her work and dedication to the Esophageal Cancer Support Group.

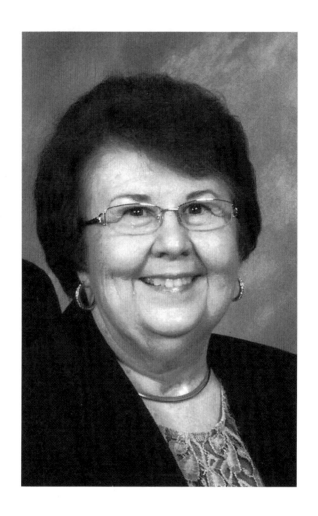

Clare L.

Chapter 4

Know That Life Is A Gift

by Clare L.

My journey began during a routine check-up with my primary care doctor. I mentioned the post-eating discomfort and the occasional vomiting I was experiencing. (I found out later that these symptoms were not caused from the cancer but rather a non-sliding hiatal hernia.) My doctor suggested having an endoscope as I suffered from acid reflux and had been on GERD (Gastroesophageal Reflux Disease) medications for probably fifteen years, and it was about six years since my last scope. I scheduled the scope, and for the first time ever since having scopes, the doctor told me he removed a small polyp and would send it away for testing. He told me that I should not worry, and that it looked ok to him.

On Sunday, December 10, 2009, I received a call from the gastroenterologist saying that he was terribly sorry. He proceeded to inform me that the results were positive, and I indeed had esophageal cancer. He instructed me to call his office in the morning and set up appointments for scans and surgeons.

"Ok, I have cancer, now what?" I thought. Being told you have cancer sets your world spinning out of control, and part of me was now numb. I had so many questions, and I knew I only had one chance to beat this. It had to be the best chance I could find. Needless to say, instead of getting ready for Christmas, I was now faced with many decisions to make with this horrifying diagnosis. Telling my children was the hardest part as I did not want them to worry. I thought to myself, "How can this be? I feel ok. I am sixty-three years old and married with three grown children and eight young grandchildren. I have so much to live for."

One of the first things I did was pray for guidance and direction. I then went online and started reading about esophageal cancer.

Unfortunately, I found the statistics on surviving esophageal cancer are not good.

The next couple of weeks were extremely busy with tests and doctors' appointments. I did not feel comfortable with the surgical procedure at the hospital I was at, so I started questioning another opinion. I wanted that 'Get Out Of Cancer Free Card' and knew I needed to be treated at the best possible facility.

I contacted an acquaintance, a doctor in the cancer research field from Canada whom my husband and I had met on a cruise years ago. I told him I had an appointment at MD Anderson Cancer Center in Texas because I wanted to get the best treatment I could and that I had read many favorable reports on the facility. He told me they were good but not to overlook the great hospital in my own backyard, the University of Michigan Health System. After talking with my oncologist (who was not a U-M doctor), he also recommended the University of Michigan Health System because they had a doctor who pioneered a surgery there for this specific type of cancer.

Further research on the internet led me to Dr. Mark Orringer. I called his office and was encouraged to go to the esophageal cancer support group meeting that week. My husband and I went and I knew then that I was in the right place. Seeing people who had been through what I was facing, looking healthy, and living normal lives, gave me the hope I needed. I brought all my tests and scan reports with me and gave them to the nurse, Lori, that evening. A few days later I received a call saying that Dr. Orringer would take me as a patient. I had my initial appointment, and after that I have never looked back. After my first appointment, I was in survivor mode and began the recommended walking three miles a day and using the spirometer. I was determined to be in the best physical shape possible to face this surgery.

I had the usual PET scan, which showed some other "spots". I was told that everyone has spots that show up on this scan and that I should not worry. My spots were mainly on the thyroid and kidneys. The spots on the thyroid bothered me the most as they were brighter.

After my constant prodding, my oncologist agreed to have a biopsy of the thyroid. More devastating news came my way. I had thyroid cancer, too, on both sides of the thyroid gland.

I was extremely anxious before surgery, and I couldn't wait to get the cancer out of me. I knew I was in great hands. I had prayed a lot and placed my trust in God and the doctors. I thought, "Whatever this is, I'll deal with it," as I hoped for the best. I was fortunate that I was in Stage I for the esophageal cancer and needed no additional treatments except for the surgery, which was scheduled for March 17, 2010. I was going to have the thyroid removed first by Dr. Barbara M., and then Dr. Mark Orringer would perform the transhiatal esophagectomy the same day.

My surgery didn't go perfectly. I developed a bleed and had to have a thoracotomy performed, which resulted in the loss of a couple pints of blood. Recovery was slow for me as well. I was in the hospital for thirty-one days instead of the seven to ten days originally thought. I had complications of a leak in the back of the anastomosis, which required a surgery and left an open wound in my neck that required packing.

I then developed an infection and they had to open the abdominal incision, which required another surgery with a 'wound vac' put in for faster healing. Both open wounds required packing and several weeks of home care from visiting nurses. I also developed blood clots in both legs and pneumonia - just some minor setbacks. I only mention these complications because there are some of us who fall in the two percent who suffer side effects; however, the body can heal and come through more than you think. It is what it is, and you have to get up each day and do what you have to do to get better. The main thing was that the esophageal cancer was contained and had not spread.

The thyroid cancer was a little worse than first thought being at Stage II, which required radioactive iodine treatments. Fortunately, both cancers have stayed in remission, and I am enjoying and living life normally. I suffer from some of the normal side effects from the surgery, but they have not stopped me from living and enjoying my life.

In the beginning, I needed stretching of my throat a few times as swallowing became difficult, but luckily I haven't had any problems for three years now. I can swallow well. I sleep elevated on a couple of pillows, and I avoid sugar as it seems to bother me; however, there are many substitutes one can use. I can eat almost anything. I just have to remind myself to eat slowly and not to overeat; otherwise, I am miserable for the next hour. I enjoy my times with family and especially my grandchildren. My husband and I travel, go on cruises, and we just recently bought a new motor home and look forward to spending a summer in Alaska.

I feel the care I received during my stay at the University of Michigan Health System was exemplary. Their nurses and physician assistants know what they are doing. They deal with this type of surgery every day. It is not a procedure that they only encounter a few times a year. Recovery takes time, and you have to be patient. However, it does get better. In the first year every new month brings added normalcy to your life. It just takes time.

Because of the open abdominal incision, I developed an incisional hernia that required surgery a year later where mesh was put in for an abdominal wall reconstruction. So I guess I can say it took me over a year to really get back my strength and feel "normal" again. But now, after three and one-half years, I can honestly say I feel well and appreciate my life.

My faith and trust in God were a vital part of getting me through this journey as well as the blessings of much love and support from my family and friends. I know this is a very serious disease. I have seen it come back to some who have gone through much more than I have and eventually claim their lives.

There are no guarantees in life, but I feel I had the best chance of beating this at the University of Michigan Health System. Dr. Orringer and his team consistently do an amazing job and put their whole lives into their work. I am forever grateful to him and all who have aided in my recovery. Live your life every day, and know that life is a gift. Be grateful for each and every day.

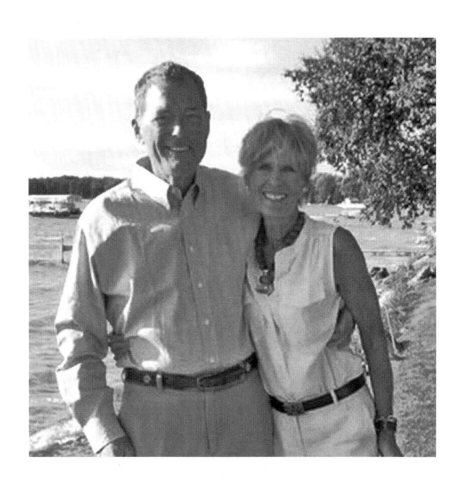

Bob and Connie L.

Chapter 5

Tales From The Blindside

by Connie L.

"Between stimulus and response there is space. In that
space is our power to choose our response. In our
response lies our growth and our freedom."
Viktor Frankl, "*Man's Search for Meaning*"

During the summer of 2011 the difficulty I experienced swallowing
was increasing. I did my best to conceal this condition but my family
(daughter Amanda was living with us at the time) was getting
suspicious. In a weird coincidence, my dentist was to work on a
crown the day before my scheduled colonoscopy/endoscopy but
could not get the Novocain to numb me sufficiently, so the
procedure was postponed. Had he been able to give me the
temporary crown, my endoscopy would have been cancelled.

One Sunday, around the same time, our substitute minister gave a
short homily on the freedom to choose fear or faith. I paid close
attention to this message, applying the theory to my putting stroke.
In the coming months I learned to appreciate the larger aspects of
the ability to choose.

These and other little signals and coincidences have played a major
part in my recovery.

Excerpts from emails and journal entries

August 10, 2011
Because of some history of swallowing difficulty, I elected to have an
endoscopy while undergoing a routine colonoscopy at Moore
Regional Hospital, Pinehurst, North Carolina. The doctor was
startled to report that the endoscopy revealed my esophagus was so
damaged it appeared to be shredded, "as though drinking lye". A
small tumor was detected and dilation was performed.

August 28, 2011
A follow-up endoscopy showed that the constriction recurred; another biopsy was performed to investigate further.

October 1, 2011
I was ordered to have a test called a barium swallow. Anything with the word "swallow" involved was cause for high anxiety. I recalled that my granddaughter, Hadley, at age ten days took the stuff down from a bottle without a flinch. She gave me courage. The test was not painful.

October 14, 2011
All the data from various tests revealed possible cancer of my esophagus with surgery recommended. Causes were unclear but the damage was obvious and the remedy would be pretty radical. Scarlett invited me to ride with her to Chapel Hill for her annual check after kidney cancer. That day she showed me the ins and outs of parking, registration and logistics. We laughed and cried together and provided moral support at both ends of the cancer spectrum.

Bob has spent three days cleaning the garage, the yard, the pool, and the car - literally everything with a hard surface. Tracy has threatened to bring her car over for detailing. This is the way we deal with fear and stress around here. We get busy.

October 17, 2011
My first appointment with my new internist. Between the time I scheduled this 'routine' appointment and the time I presented, the game had changed dramatically. To prepare for the challenges ahead he ordered an x-ray, respiratory, and blood tests. We laid the groundwork for the doctors ahead. All test reports showed excellent results. No problem!

October 21, 2011
My first meeting with the team at UNC. I had an ultrasound and Endoscopic mucosal resection in an attempt to remove the tumor located against my vocal chords. The tumor could not be removed because it was not stable. The diagnosis was still not clear so lots of

scraping and photos occurred. Many of the UNC specialists were called in to have a look. A very unusual case.

October 26, 2011
Kathleen, P.A., reported the results of the ultrasound as not cancer but virus. This diagnosis was later rejected and cancer was confirmed. The recommendation is immediate esophagectomy. PET and CT scans scheduled.

October 28, 2011
I am admitted to Women's Hospital at UNC for PET scan, CT scan and consultation. The process is very calm, quiet and professional. The staff is careful to be sure I am warm and comfortable. The kindness of all the caregivers makes this almost a religious experience. Very quiet. I meditate, 100, 99, 98........

Dr. V. confirms that this is indeed cancer, no question. Remedy is again - no question - esophagectomy. The pathology showed the tumor is stage 1 cancer, no radiation or chemo recommended at this time. We are encouraged to get a second opinion and Dr. Mark Orringer, chief of Thoracic Surgery, University of Michigan Hospital is the natural selection. Dr. Orringer had been introduced to us by Mike and also was known to us as the surgeon for our friend Terry in 1990.

With so much to accept and contemplate, we drive quietly home until we had a blowout on Hwy 1. Perfect.

October 27, 2011
Attend the UNC football game and tailgate with Debbie and Spike. A wonderful day.

October 28, 2011
Spend a great afternoon with the gun club trying to blow up the clay pigeons.

> Date: October 29, 2011
> Email from: Connie
>
> Hi, All. Here is the scoop…wow, this is tough to write.

Yesterday the doctors at UNC confirmed that I have esophageal cancer. This diagnosis is the result of two endoscopies, an endoscopic ultrasound, PET scan, and CT scan. I had been experiencing some difficulty swallowing certain food for about six months.

The good news that comes with this is that the cancer is confined to my esophagus and may be rather new. I feel fine and the doctors expect a full recovery without chemo/radiation. They think I am tough enough to make them look good.

So here is the plan. Bob and I are preparing for surgery at UNC to remove my esophagus. We have met with the surgeon and will be traveling to the University of Michigan to visit with the specialist there for a second opinion. Apparently, this type of cancer is extremely rare, so all the doctors are buddies and discuss techniques and procedures with each other. If, as we expect, all the opinions are confirmed, I will have this done the first week in December.

Between now and then, I am going to train like I am in a marathon to prepare my body, get my Christmas shopping done, and play as much golf as I can. I am also supposed to keep my weight up so anytime you want to go out for lunch or dinner… I know you have all been keeping a vigil with us and we have come to rely on your prayers and support. Please don't stop now.

It seems unbelievably strange to report this to you because I feel so well. I will see all of you at the golf course, the poker table, or the dinner table, so keep in touch.
XOX
Connie

November 7, 2011
Bob and I meet with Dr. Orringer at 8:00am at the University of Michigan Hospital. He spends an hour with us explaining esophageal cancer and his recommended surgery for esophagectomy. He is modest, calm and very confident. He carefully explains the special technique required due to the location of the tumor. He describes

how he will tweak this and tease that so that when I awake from surgery I can say "this sucks" and he will be able to hear me.

We are anxious to have this surgery immediately and move on with our lives. Another intervention occurs. Dr. Orringer is unable to perform my surgery until 1/10 due to his travel and teaching schedule. I ask what I could do to prepare. I get a spirometer to use every day and instructions to walk three miles every day. My training begins. I believe this ultimately saved my life.

November 16, 2011
Dr. V. and I discuss by phone the various recommendations before us regarding esophagectomy. The decision is remarkably easy. Dr. V. advises us to go to Michigan for surgery with Dr. Orringer. Dr. V. is not feeling confident in his ability for this delicate situation. Dr. V. has performed about 250 such surgeries and Dr. Orringer had 3,000 under his scalpel the week we visited him.

November 17, 2011 – January 6, 2012
Bob and I concentrate on making the most of each day and each situation. We say yes to each invitation to play golf, bridge or have dinner. We receive with gratitude all of the offers of prayer and support and gain a sense of wellbeing for its own sake. To be sure, we experience the fear and apprehension of an unknown future but we try not to inflict each other and others with the tension this creates. We make our travel plans, follow the doctors' orders, and pay our bills. We have a bunch of family and pals for Thanksgiving and Christmas. We walk the dogs, enjoy our cocktail hour and listen with care to the sound advice of our friends. Late one cold afternoon, my girlfriends arrived for a "surgery shower". They gift me with the slippers, heating pads, books and blankets required for a long recovery. That day, nurse Bob administered Cosmos. Standing in Susie and Gus's kitchen one evening feeling the pressure, Adair reminds me that I should not let my imagination get ahead of my reality. Excellent advice. I am practicing this theory.

During this time, Sam, the "minister of putting", came into our circle of friends. Knowing, but not knowing that we needed spiritual support, we made a date for Sam to visit for tea. Drinking tea in the afternoon has never been a part of our life and sharing our personal fears even less so. Sam makes it easy for us. We get acquainted and know that when needed, he will be ready to step in. This we can do. Sam talks about the women's basketball coach from Tennessee State. With regard to her recent cancer diagnosis she said, "It is what it is. What it becomes is up to me."

January 6, 2012
Bob and I take the long drive through the snow to Michigan. We are the only people on the road heading North at this time of the year. In spite of the miserable trip and the trepidation we experience, we know for sure we have made the right choices all along. This helps. Through the kindness of Susie and Mike, Bob and I are invited to stay in the house of their friends, Dede and Jim, while we are in Ann Arbor. The house is great and Mike and Susie are down the road. We unpack and quietly wait for January 10.

January 9, 2012
Dr. Orringer's nurse, Lori Flint, calls to advise that Dr. Orringer has had a personal emergency and cannot take me on January 10th. The good news is she called just before I drank the "cleanser". The bad news is she is not sure when I can get in. This is probably the worst news we have yet received. Later, we are told that we will be delayed only one day. This helps us keep our mental momentum flowing.

January 11, 2012
Bob and I arrive at U-M at 5:30am. From this point the story gets sketchy. Surgery takes six and one-half hours. The procedure is relatively routine, the exception being the tumor location causing Dr. Orringer to cut through the sphincter and leaving only a tiny bit to attach my stomach to the remaining tissue. Hand sewing rather than staples cause a more fragile anastomosis. But the job is complete and I am sent to my room with nine tubes connecting me to an IV pole.

Nursing care is around the clock for the first 24 hours. Dr. Orringer's physician assistant is stationed across the hall and watchful. The first three days I am encouraged to walk the halls pushing the IV with all the apparatus as much as possible. I have ice and water and began clear liquids on the fourth day. I am able to take care of myself getting up and down and am quite mobile. I attribute this to all the physical training.

The pain is in the form of a headache, likely the result of the epidural. I had experienced this once before when Amanda was born - same drug. My body mends very well but the headache continues.

Day 5 post-op, I get rid of some of the tubes. The chest tubes are the most painful both in and upon removal. They are big tubes and I am relatively small so I feel the compression. I have had the good fortune to be cared for by wonderful nurses. Melissa has taken me under her wing and supervises the others (should I say 'bossed'?), in the delicate aspects of my care. All the nurses will leave this work behind to return home to full-on family obligations. I do not know how they have so much to give.

I am released from U-M on the 8th day.

> Date: January 11, 2012
> Email from: Bob
>
> GREAT NEWS!!! Our girl came through today and knocked it out of the park. She went into the operating room at 7:30. As she was wheeled out, the pre-op nurse looked at me and said, "You lose." Her blood pressure was 102 over 72 – almost comatose. Connie had told the nurse that she and I always have this contest over who has the lowest blood pressure. Can you believe she went into this operation with that B/P? Mine would have been 190/120. The operation was supposed to last seven hours, and she was out in six. The Dr., who is not very effusive, came out and said he couldn't be happier with the results, nor could I !! One of the main worries was the proximity of the tumor to the voice box.
>
> When I walked into the recovery room, Sweet Con looked up and said in a great voice, "How are you?" I said, "You have a voice." She said, "Sure." We have a few more things to get through, but this is a great first step. I will see her the first thing next morning. Hopefully, she will have a peaceful night's sleep.

Thank you very much for all your prayers. I am sure that God does listen.

Bob

Date: January 12, 2012
Email from: Bob

Everyone, the first night was not exactly as we wanted. Connie was allergic to the epidural sedative, and her blood pressure went down to 40/20 – not good. They changed the meds to a high-powered Motrin, and she is doing great. Let me just say to see her makes me want to cringe; she has nine tubes in her right now. What a tough lady. They will all stay until Saturday when, hopefully, six will be removed. She got up and walked the halls four times today, tubes and all. Not far, but four times. Tomorrow is her 67th birthday. Friday the 13th – can you believe that? I am absolutely sure my report will be much more upbeat tomorrow.

We love you all.

Bob

January 18, 2012
Bob and I are staying in the home of Loretta and Jim for recovery. Jill provides professional nurses for the night and Nurse Bob is on the day shift. I am instructed to eat a mushy diet but food tasted really, really awful. Nothing tastes as I expect or remember. Chef Bob is very frustrated and tries hard to entice me. I force what is possible and rely on the feeding tube. My headache is persistent but otherwise I am improving. Bob administers all the meds with real expertise. We have drugs and supplies everywhere. It is incredibly nice to be in this beautiful home with a fire and friends.

Date: January 21, 2012
Email from: Connie

Hi, All. Today is what is known in the medical field as 'Patient Day 10'. This is a red-letter day. There are several along the way. Day 3 means some of the various tubes are removed, easing the burden on the IV pole. Day 5 I can't remember because I felt so shitty. However, this is Day 10! That means that danger is behind, the medications are beginning to do their advance work and I am definitely coming out of the woods.

You will see from the photo taken from the front door that Michigan is beautiful today. I walked this morning and Bob and I are due for another round in about an hour. It has been great to see our old pals and they are kicking in with love, soup, and support. Mary P. came yesterday to whip my hair into shape. The kindness of all of you continues to overwhelm us with gratitude. Believe me, when you catch a cold, I will be the first one on your doorstep.

We will hang here a few more days. On Thursday we will visit the magician that performed this surgery for the release to leave the state. We are expecting to return next weekend. Amazing, I think. One little note about Bobby L. Has he not been incredible? He takes care of all the details, makes the medicine go down and buys everything he walks by to cheer me up.

This has been a weird and beautiful blessing.

XO
C

January 25, 2012
We visit with Dr. Orringer to be released for home. I have a slight temp and headache. Dr. Orringer dilates my throat, or tries to anyway. This might be the corollary to waterboarding. It is awful. Given my history of swallowing issues the sight of the bougie device freaks me out. Once done, Dr. Orringer signs the papers and we are free to travel. Then, the shit hits the fan.

January 27, 2012
Bob leaves at 5:00am for the twelve-hour drive to NC. John and Julia are due to fly up here in the afternoon, spend the night with me and fly me home Saturday morning. Adriane and Del are coming with dinner for all of us. How unbelievably generous are our friends.

As the morning progresses my temperature rises and the headache continues. Erica comes at 1:00 to give me a massage. She comes regularly to help circulation and keep the medications moving through my system and out. I am starting to realize I am really sick. I contact John and Julia while they were still at the NC airport to delay their departure while I figure out what to do.

By 3:00 I am certain I cannot leave Michigan. I wait until about 3:30 to call Bob and tell him the bad news. He might turn the car around and come back to Michigan. That is too much and too dangerous in the snow and stress. Adriane and Del come with dinner and Adriane brings along her nightclothes to stay with me. How does she know when I don't that this will be so prophetic?

> Date: January 27, 2012
> Email from: Bob
>
> Shit happens!! I left B'ham this morning at 5:00, expecting C to follow with friends tomorrow. That's not happening. Con woke up with a temp and Dr. O. didn't want her to leave. She didn't call me and tell me this until she knew I was in NC and couldn't turn around. Very sneaky. We don't think this is very much, but you never know. Mandy is with me tonight and that is great. I am not sure what is going to happen the next few days, but I will keep you informed. Bo just came up and put his head on my lap. What could be better?
>
> Bob

January 28, 2012 3:00am
I call Dr. Orringer's physician assistant on duty and report my temp at 103. I have to go back to the hospital. Adriane and I find our way through a snowstorm to the hospital where the emergency people are waiting for me. Thank you, Ron. I am admitted smoothly. I can't let Adriane call Bob until about 7:30. He is exhausted from the drive home and must rest. There is surely more to come. I am safe and in very good hands. I am not afraid.

January 28, 2012
By midafternoon, Bob is back in my room. I am so grateful. I have symptoms of pneumonia, my headache is raging. Other than that, I feel pretty okay. I am admitted and under observation by the physician assistants. Dr. Orringer is in Florida attending a

conference. I have a barium swallow and the radiologist thinks it is okay. Amy, physician assistant, smells a rat. All day she has been hovering, fretting, wondering what is going on with me. Finally, she reviews the barium test with Bob. By now, Bob is up to speed on all procedures and confident to give an opinion. On the screen there is a faint detection of a "swoosh" on the swallow test. There is a leak in the anastomosis and bacteria are being released into my system. Amy and Bob know this. They are sure of this.

Date: January 29, 2012
Email from: Bob

To all - I just found the cord to the computer to charge it. I am a spastic. Well, two nights ago Connie got worse. Thank God Adriane D. was staying with her. Con woke up at 3:00 feeling like crap. At 3:30, in a blizzard, they left for the hospital. When they got to Ann Arbor, they started a myriad of tests – great place. Adriane said at one point they took C to have a chest x-ray and said, "We'll be back in five minutes". In five minutes C was back. Adriane called me with this development around 7:30. I had to find a place for the dogs, Gus and Susie L. As Gus said, "Why not have six?" Thank you, Gus and Susie!

I got a plane at 12:40 out of Raleigh and was in Connie's room at 4:30. The one thing that was for sure was that the white blood count was high, meaning it was trying to fight an infection somewhere. Their best guess right now is that it is a bladder infection. If there had to be an infection, bladder is the best – easiest to control. However, the damn headache is still there and throbbing. Seventeen days. We hope this is just a little ding in our door and will be coming home soon. Will keep you all informed.

Bob

January 30, 2012
Dr. Lin is called in. Amy tells Bob to go home to Birmingham and rest. This will take a while. I am calm, not in pain, and full of faith that this will turn out well. In fact, what is taking Dr. Lin so long? Let's go. Dr. Lin repairs the tear in the anastomoses. He also discovers a blood clot in my jugular vein.

I awake in a magical place. Danielle, the most beautiful blond nurse, is taking care of me. Am I dead? I must be. My headache is gone. Bob is here. I know, I know that all will be well. Danielle bathes me and washes my hair. It is reverent. Bob is sleeping in the next room. I feel levitated, transformed.

Date: January 31, 2012
Email from: Bob

Last night I got a call from the hospital that C was in ICU after the operation. So, off I went, back to Ann Arbor, and talked my way into ICU at around midnight. There I saw this really great nurse taking care of Connie – everything she needed. The operation went better than expected. The incision on the neck was re-opened and they found a rather large hole in the connection to the stomach. The incision was not sealed and will be left open to heal from the inside out.

She does have a pneumonia, which they are aggressively fighting with antibiotics. Now, the good news. The intern came in about 5:30 (when do they sleep?) and said all looks really good. He asked how Con felt and she said, "GREAT". Can you imagine having a five-inch open slice in your neck and saying, "Great"? She is one tough lady. I know she is feeling better; no headaches at all – first time in eighteen days. Bob

January 30, 2012
Alex arrives. I am still in ICU and Bill is my new nurse. He is full of joy and good will. I feel wonderful but Alex is sure I am going to die. He thinks I look awful. He does not know. This is the beginning of my recovery. I have pneumonia and blood poisoning, but I do not have a headache. I will be well.

February 1, 2012
Dr. Orringer has returned with a vengeance. Late evening he has come to check on me. The anastomosis is healing perfectly now, from the inside out. Now, we are aggressively fighting pneumonia. The antibiotics are fighting blood poisoning; Bob is being trained by Amy in the art of wound care. Bob does not flinch. He cleans, swabs, and disinfects the anastomosis site, places the dressing just so,

and pretends he does not see the tears rolling down my cheeks. He is not hurting me, I just can't believe he can do this. Mandy arrives. In our attempt to maintain perspective, we held our children off a little bit. We have done them a disservice. Their presence gives us comfort we realize we desperately need.

February 2, 2012
My feeding tube is reinstalled. This is a major accomplishment because it had been out for the maximum amount of time and scar tissue was quickly forming. Dr. Orringer had 'tagged' the site, which made this procedure successful. I am wheeled into the most beautiful, brand new surgery. Right out of a movie set for nuclear medicine for the 22nd century.

Date: February 03, 2012
Email from: Bob

Well, sports fans, the hits just keep on coming. Dr. O. saw Connie last night and confirmed that the lung problem is ARDS, acute respiratory distress syndrome – not pneumonia. ARDS is a very different problem. It is not affected by any antibiotics. It is only cured by the person's own body. Thank God Connie is so strong. Her white blood count is still elevated, which means there is still an infection somewhere, which they are working diligently to find. HOWEVER, I just talked to Connie and she sounded GREAT!!! Mandy is coming in from Charlotte today as a little surprise for Connie. She will love it. We will talk tonight.
Bob

Date: February 4, 2012
Email from: Bob

To all. It is a wonder what a Mother's children can do. First Alex and today Mandy. Both times she saw her children, you could see the will and love strengthen in Connie's eyes. We also had a long talk with Dr. O. We are not getting out soon, but Con is definitely doing MUCH better. Another milestone, nurse Bob changed the dressing on "patient's" neck. It was a piece of cake – not! And, I will be having a larger vodka this evening. See you tomorrow.

NB

February 9, 2012

Back to R's home for the final lap. I have lost about twenty pounds - from 124 - and Nurse Bob is again trying to get me to eat. Food tastes disgusting but I am trying. I now love and respect my little feeding tube. This is a device to embrace. There is nothing to it and it makes you feel good. My wonderful nurses return at night to give us both the peaceful rest we need. Nurse Bob takes care of my wound very professionally. We have a very funny (not funny) encounter with a visiting nurse. Hire a private if you possibly can. It did not take Nurse Bob long to kick her out. That is another story.

Date: February 11, 2012
Email from: Connie

Hi, All. It is lovely to be in Birmingham and out of the hospital. We have a foot of snow and the sun is shining. I am tucked in by a fire and getting ready for a snooze. Not too bad.

As Bob has reported, the last couple of weeks have been crazy. Fortunately, I do not really remember too much of the details. I just kind of floated along on the prayers and support you all were sending hourly. I am really improving each day now. No aches or pains, just a little thin. I will come back quickly with the smell and beauty of home and the ability to get outside and walk.

It looks like we will be able to break for home next Saturday. We can barely wait.

Last night, a home health nurse was sent by some Medicare provider to check me out, etc. Fortunately, we had a private nurse standing by to watch and help us through an IV hookup, etc. So, this Medicare nurse comes in, all disorganized and really none too clean or inspiring. She starts a pitch about her company, yada yada, and we are looking at her like "is she nuts?." Really, do we care? Then she starts to sneeze and blow her nose, grabbing the closest paper towel to wipe up. We are trying to back out of the room. Finally, Bob blows! He kicked her out! Honestly, it was hilarious. Bobby L. does it again.

We will let you know what happens next. Thanks for all the cards and emails. We so love hearing from all of you.

XO, C

February 16, 2012
Back to U-M for the final reports. We are on our way home!

February 17, 2012
Alex, Meredith and our grandchildren, Kate, Hadley and Jack visit us. The little ones cannot detect the importance of their visit. But for Bob and me it is the culmination of the work we have done over the last weeks. Pay day. Our visit is completely ordinary, easy, and nothing special, everything is okay. No apprehension in the grandchildren, no anxiety in the adults. Love you, see you soon!

Dave and Paula offer their plane for our return to NC. We recognize the importance of this and are grateful, once again, for the kindness of our friends. Paying forward the kindness we have accepted will be our intention in the years to come.

By Saturday afternoon when we arrive home, all the support supplies are here as well. I have an IV pole, nutrition, and oxygen by 5:00pm. Bob has a cocktail by 6:00. I am in heaven by 7:00.

February 19, 2012 – March 31, 2012
The gentle work of recuperation is beginning. I feel well but pretty weak. But each day I see a little improvement. I can walk the dogs a short way, play bridge, visit with friends. I am weaning myself from the feeding tube, which initially took 14 hours a day. Naps are shorter. My anastomosis is forming scar tissue at a very rapid rate. I returned to UNC for after-care and regular endoscopies to stretch my throat. It is still quite difficult to swallow. I am now making friends with the staff in the GI unit. I am begging them for their tee shirt. It says UNC – GI Right on Track. Pretty cute.

April 1, 2012 – December 1, 2012
I have gained some weight and like my new body. I play golf and travel. My energy level and strength still are somewhat retarded. I can eat almost anything but still return to UNC for periodic

endoscopies to stretch my throat. Dr. Orringer told me that I can do much better and has encouraged me to attempt self-dilation. I have the sense that I've let him down and vow to work on it, sometime…..

December 16, 2012
Brian, our physician friend and neighbor has agreed to be my dilation coach. In an email he actually said, "Gulp". Very funny guy. Sunday afternoon he arrives with his bundle of bougies slung over his shoulder and a bottle of Lidocaine. Together, we try to coax that device down my throat. Forty-five minutes later, in full sweat, we decide to try it again the following Sunday. His Zen approach to the procedure helps me breathe and visualize what needs to happen. It is rough and unsuccessful but it is a start and I slowly began to overcome my fear.

January 1, 2013
Brian has allowed me to keep a 24cc bougie and practice on my own. Every morning I take it down and hold it for 30 seconds. I feel my courage increase each time. I am now in control of the device and more important, I am in control of my body.

January 11, 2013
Bob and I are sailing in the British Virgin Islands. Hard to believe. I am wearing a bikini and feel wonderful.

February 1, 2013 - March 1, 2013
Bob and I spend the month in Naples, FL. I begin to work out every day. Kick boxing, yoga, weight training, whatever the gym puts in front of me. Every morning I dilate my throat for 30 seconds. I am now up to 34 French and on my way to 42. That is the goal Dr. Orringer has set for me. I can do it. I walk the dogs three miles most days and play lots of golf. I look for ways to repay all the kindness given to me.

> "If you need me to
> Take your hand and pull you through,
> Friends like you there are too few, just one or two
> I will remember you"
Bobby Runk, "*I Will Remember You*".

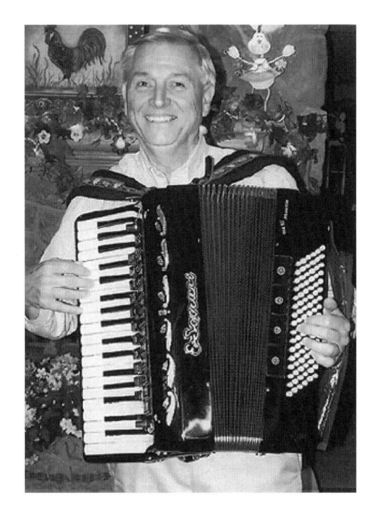

John K.

Chapter 6

My Path To Surviving And Thriving

by John K.

My story began back in July of 2002 when I had a routine physical exam and the blood work indicated I had a low red blood cell count and my primary care physician in Gaylord, Michigan asked me to at least have an upper GI; the results of which displayed a lesion. He immediately referred me to a gastroenterologist in Petoskey who, after he saw the x-rays, asked if I could stay long enough for him to scope my esophagus, which I did. The bad news was the photo of the cancer at the opening to my stomach. The good news was that it was discovered early enough to be operable. Of course, he contacted my referring doctor and as soon as he got the information he referred me to the University of Michigan, Thoracic Surgery Department.

My first meeting there was with Dr. John Yee who had all of my records. He concluded that it would be wise to have the transhiatal esophagectomy, and he recommended that I receive radiation and chemotherapy before the surgery. He, along with an oncologist in Petoskey, designed the protocol that I should take; five weeks of radiation on a daily basis - Monday through Friday - and chemotherapy infusions in the Northern Michigan Hospital, full-time on the first and fifth week of the radiation treatments. The infusions were to last 96 hours each time I was in the hospital. Once that was done, which was near the end of October, 2002, I was scheduled for my operation on November 11, 2002.

I was in the hospital for 10 days due the fact that I am diabetic and the healing process did take a little longer. I was discharged on November 20, 2002 and my wife (who was driving) and I stopped at a Cracker Barrel restaurant on the way back to my home in Gaylord. I had a meatloaf meal along with the fixings and although I couldn't eat much of it, I had no ill effects. I then began the recovery process at home.

37

When Thanksgiving Day arrived my wife drove me to Empire, Michigan, which is a few miles west of Traverse City, to have dinner with close friends. That is where I had my first dumping issue, which occurred right after I ate some cranberry sauce. The sugar did me in. Fortunately, one of the other guests at the meal was a nurse and she recognized my agony right away and helped me endure this first episode with cold packs and getting me into a reclining position with my head elevated.

I returned to my work as a bank president by December 15, 2002 and attended our company Christmas party for an abbreviated amount of time. When I got home I suffered another bout with dumping, probably because I ate too much. I quickly learned that foods that are high in fats and sugars offer the potential of dumping, so that now I completely avoid them most of the time.

I drove to Ann Arbor by myself for follow up visits with Dr. Yee on a quarterly basis three times and had no difficulty in doing that. In April of 2003, I got my boat out of storage and towed it to Anna Maria Island, Florida, where I had rented a house for a month. The Chairman of my Bank Board had a place there and invited me to join him for an Easter meal, which I did without incident. However, at that gathering I asked if we could come up with a way for me to retire early. He and the Board put together a very generous package that allowed me to do just that.

In August of 2003, my mother who lived in Brighton, Michigan was in failing health due to ovarian cancer. So, I sold my house in Gaylord and moved to Hartland, MI to be able to help her get to where she needed to go for her numerous doctor appointments and hospital visits.

By this time my wife was saying that I was much too young to be retired so I went to work for a large mortgage company as a Regional Builder Manager, covering three states, Michigan, Wisconsin, and Minnesota. That job meant that I was meeting with homebuilders and developers involving a lot of travel, which I tolerated very well and enjoyed immensely. The mortgage business, as you know, collapsed in 2007 and the Builder Manager Department was shut down in August. Shortly afterward my mom passed away.

In September I began to work in Ann Arbor for an old friend who had started a leasing company, and I am doing that as we speak. It's a sales job that requires only phone contacts, but when added to my other activities, it keeps me quite busy. I mention all of this because folks who are contemplating this kind of surgery, chemotherapy and radiation need to know that life can go on at a high level of activity. The only real issue that one has to deal with, in my opinion, is learning what and how to eat and, of course, how best to sleep.

As I mentioned, I am diabetic (Type II) and during the time that I was being radiated and infused with chemotherapy I was insulin dependent. Dr. Yee predicted that three months after my surgery I would in all likelihood lose about 30% of my body weight and would no longer be insulin dependent. That has proven to be the case. While I still monitor my blood sugar and am taking small quantities of oral medication, again I am doing quite well. I regularly visit a new primary care physician and he, too, is happy to see how well I do as compared to his other patients my age, which is now 70.

Although the circumstances for having a dumping event are now greatly diminished because I have learned what my body can tolerate, I still make a mistake once in a while by eating either too much or food with a high fat or sugar content. I have never had a problem with seafood, chicken or vegetables and can drink milk and an occasional beer or cocktail. To jump-start my taste buds after the surgery, I discovered that eating spicy foods did the trick, i.e. blackened broiled fish or spicy seafood. I also found that sour foods like dill pickles and sauerkraut helped. To this day I love to eat both of them - without incident.

As we all learn after the surgery, the nerve that controls acid no longer works as it has been severed. But bile continues to be produced and if it refluxes while you are sleeping, it is a very bad experience. The result is that I have to sleep with my head elevated, which is the case with most of us who have had the surgery.

With all of this being the case, I have stated many times that I would undergo what I have done over again without any hesitation. First, the procedure - while complex - is something that one can survive. You cannot survive this cancer; it is far too deadly. Second, I made the right choice of where and who should manage what had to be done; the U-M Hospital. Its dedicated team has years of experience in the treatment of esophageal cancer and surgeries that are often used as a cure. Finally, the support group that has been led by Lori Flint is the only place where all of the issues regarding pre- and post-surgery are openly discussed.

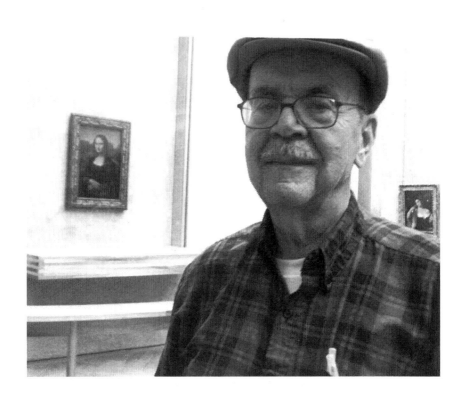

Ken S.

Chapter 7

Each New Day Is A Blessing

by Ken S.

Ten years ago (2005) I was diagnosed with Stage III esophageal cancer and given twelve months to live. Two years earlier (2003) after thirty-six years as an archivist at the University of Michigan, I retired to the area near Cincinnati, Ohio, where most of my family lived and where my mother resided in assisted living. Upon receiving my cancer diagnosis, at the urging of friends, I returned to Ann Arbor for my surgery and follow-up treatment by Dr. Orringer, without whom I never would have made it.

Although I never married, I had strong kinship and friendship ties which proved of great help in battling cancer. In 1937 I was born to a working class family in Mt. Healthy, Ohio (then a small town, now a suburb of Cincinnati). My father was a truck driver and factory worker. My mother was the matriarch of her family as her mother had been before her. During the midst of the Depression, my maternal grandfather lingered with colon cancer for five years, and my mother, being the oldest able-bodied of his children, sacrificed her dream of an education, lied about her age, and went to work to support the family. So while I was an only child, I had cousins who were like brothers and sisters to me.

Like other members of my family, I also developed strong friendships. My maternal grandmother, an Irish-American cleaning lady, had what we called 'the gift of gab.' She was friendly and sociable (as was my dad); traits she transmitted to her children. And she taught me an important lesson early, saying, "What goes around comes around" (i.e., the way you treat others is the way you will be treated). It certainly benefited her for she endured many hard times, and it certainly benefited me.

My swallowing problems developed a year before I was diagnosed with esophageal cancer. At my annual physical on September 1,

2004, I first told my then internist about it. When he learned that I never had heartburn, he attributed it to the normal aging process and concentrated on my growing problem with high blood pressure. On a follow-up visit nearly four months later, I told him about continuing swallowing difficulty. If it continued, he said, I should try artificial saliva, available at any pharmacy. At the time, I weighed 195 lbs., about 20 more than I should.

By my next visit (March 24, 2005) he had retired and was succeeded by a young, newly minted D.O., who specialized in gerontology. When she learned my swallowing trouble was increasing, she sent me for X-rays and a barium swallow test, which showed a narrowing of the esophagus but no tumor. So she referred me to the gastroenterologist who had been giving my family colonoscopies for years. He asked me several questions including whether I'd ever had heartburn (I hadn't). Describing my problem as 'minor' and 'easily corrected,' he scheduled me for a dilation. It showed the stricture was narrower than anticipated and I had an 'ulcer' for which he prescribed medication.

On May 24 (two days after my mom was hospitalized with congestive heart failure), I had my second EGD. My blood pressure jumped during the procedure, which my gastroenterologist reported to my internist. He found my stricture remained 'narrow' and my 'ulcer' hadn't completely healed. So he recommended drinking lots of fluids with meals, and chewing my food more thoroughly. He asked me to call him in two weeks to report how I was doing. He also took some biopsies from inside the esophagus, which proved to be negative. When my swallowing problems continued, he scheduled me for a third EGD on July 5.

In the meantime, I had my annual check-up with my dermatologist. He removed two suspicious spots on my nose, which a biopsy showed to be carcinomas. So he referred me to a specialist for more surgery (which eventually, after my esophageal diagnosis, made me feel like I was a cancer farm). Afterwards, cosmetic surgery was suggested, but I rejected it - saying I wasn't a Hollywood actor, and I'd lived for years with baldness, so I could live with a couple holes in my nose.

When I saw my internist again on June 15 I told her about my concern with my mom's health and a couple episodes of light-headedness. My vital signs were still pretty good: 168 lbs., 132/84 B.P., and 68 pulse. But she ordered an EKG, carotid artery and heart monitor tests and referred me to a cardiologist.

While I waited, I had my third EGD on July 5th. My gastroenterologist took more biopsies from inside the esophagus, which again proved negative, and ordered a CT scan, which showed a "thickening of the esophageal wall." Because of the latter, he scheduled me for an endoscopic ultrasound with his senior colleague on July 28. He told my family that he suspected esophageal cancer, which, he explained, meant I had a life expectancy of about 12 months.

In the afternoon, my cousin and his wife took me to the hospital for my esophageal ultrasound, for which I was anesthetized. Five days later, on August 2, I received the results. My gastroenterologist told me I had esophageal cancer and needed to act, "As quickly as possible." He referred me to an oncologist who squeezed me into his schedule on August 2nd - the last day before he left on vacation. That evening, I told my mom I had cancer.

The day before my oncologist appointment, I saw my internist for the last time before my treatments started. She handed me two notes to give to the oncologist. One concerned my weight loss (from 195 at the end of January to 155 today). The other said simply, "Mr. S. is an excellent patient and one of my favorite people - please let me know if I can be of assistance."

The following day, I met my oncologist. He commented that my BP reading (128/80) was excellent under the circumstances. And he told me he wanted to treat my cancer aggressively with five to six weeks each of radiation and chemotherapy (including a machine which would deliver chemo 24/7) followed by an esophagectomy. The next day, a feeding tube was installed, followed a few days later by a PET scan, and a port installation.

On August 15th my radiation and chemo treatments began. They were preceded by a meeting with both my radiologist and oncologist. My oncologist began by saying the PET scan showed that the cancer hadn't reached the lymph nodes behind the heart. So there was 'a chance' but 'no guarantee'.

I was still convinced I was going to die. After all, the gastroenterologist told my family I had twelve months to live, and my own research indicated that the five-year survival rate for esophageal cancer was about seven percent, and mine had been discovered late. I was only determined to outlive my mother because I knew how devastating the loss of her only child would be to her. As we left, the radiologist told my cousin, "If attitude can cure, this man will be cured."

As I was waiting for my first infusion, I saw a list of cancer support groups. There was none for esophageal cancer (probably because there were so few survivors), which further confirmed my belief that I was going to die. Within a couple days, radiation sealed my esophagus, so for the next three months, I was totally dependent on a feeding tube for all my nourishment.

At the end of the second week, mouth sores forced the suspension of my chemotherapy. It was resumed two times at reduced dosages, but eventually had to be stopped because of the sores. Despite them, I continued to visit my mom every day in nursing at the Christian Home. I concealed the sores with a mask, telling her it was needed to protect me from infection. The radiation continued, but the fact that I only received about 2/3 of the recommended chemo treatment further convinced me that I wasn't going to make it.

Given my belief, I began contacting as many friends as possible to say goodbye. I wanted to tell them how much I appreciated their friendship and how glad I was that they were part of my life. And I worked on tying up any loose ends which might be left in my life.

A few days after the first chemo suspension, a friend called from Ann Arbor to urge me to come there for my surgery under a Dr. Orringer, whom she claimed was "the best in the country." Other friends soon called offering places to stay for my family and me during my treatment. I told all of them that I appreciated their thoughtfulness, but I knew I was going to die and preferred to spend my remaining days close to home with my family. But the friend who initially suggested Dr. Orringer didn't give up.

She called my cousin's wife, a retired nurse, whom she knew advised me on medical matters. My Ann Arbor friend converted her by explaining the Orringer procedure. Then my relative convinced me by describing how not opening up the rib cage would make the surgery so much easier on me. So I agreed go to the U-M if Dr. Orringer would accept me as a patient.

When I first broached the possibility of having my surgery done in Michigan, my oncologist was resistant. "We have good surgeons in Cincinnati, too," he asserted. But after I mentioned Dr. Orringer's name, his attitude changed. "Oh, yes!" he said. "We give him our difficult cases. I will write him a letter. He doesn't like FAXs."

On October 11, the day after finishing my treatments in Cincinnati (and executing my estate planning documents), my cousin drove me to Michigan to meet Dr. Orringer for the first time. I noticed he had small hands but a powerful handshake. If anyone can reach under my rib cage and do the surgery, I thought, he could. He proceeded to tell us what he was going to do (making me a drawing, which I still have), why he was doing it, and what I could do to increase the chances of success, including walking three miles a day and using a breath-strengthening device. As we left, I asked him how many of these surgeries he'd done. He responded, "Over two thousand."

Six days after I returned from Ann Arbor on October 17th, my oncologist gave me an encouraging report from my last PET scan. "Now," he said, "all you need is a skilled surgeon." On my way home, I stopped at the Christian Home to tell my mom - adding that I'd see her again after lunch. Before I could return, the Home called to say she'd died of congestive heart failure. A burden was lifted from me. At least she died after receiving some good news, and she didn't have to worry about me - and me about her - while I was gone to Ann Arbor.

After Dr. Orringer reviewed my reports from Cincinnati, he asked that I see a cardiologist and have an echocardiogram. I asked my oncologist why, if I were cleared for surgery in Cincinnati, Dr. Orringer needed more information. He responded: "Dr. Orringer is very thorough."

Meanwhile, I was following Dr. Orringer's instructions religiously. This time, with my mom gone, I was just doing it for myself, but I had reason for optimism. Having survived a bout of childhood tuberculosis (in the pre-antibiotic era), I knew I didn't have the best lungs. But I was determined to do everything I could to ensure a good outcome. At my funeral I didn't want anyone to say I hadn't done my best – or that I had been a 'quitter.' And, I had my dad's example to follow. As a child, he'd survived lobar pneumonia, being hit by a car when he was five (almost being knocked into a saloon - he always said that if he'd gone through the swinging doors, his temperance parents would have disowned him), and later convulsions when his adult teeth proved too big for his mouth. So I walked at least three miles a day every day, rain or shine, except for the day I left for Ann Arbor when mid-way on my trek across my square mile home town, I saw my family gathered on my lawn to wish me goodbye.

While I'd endured serious illness as a child, I'd never had major surgery. So I asked my cousin's wife, the nurse, to accompany me and my cousin (whose daughter was named for my mom) to Ann Arbor. Unfortunately, shortly before we were scheduled to leave, her son, who was a diabetic, suffered a stroke, but a Michigan friend, who had been a nurse at University Hospital, took her place to answer any questions we might have and deal with the medical establishment for us.

On November 7, Dr. Orringer performed the esophagectomy - my first major surgery. Immediately afterwards, I returned to my room and was amazed that I had virtually no pain - only soreness. It seemingly took me all night to turn from one side to the other. Dr. Orringer visited me at least once a day during every day I was in the hospital. Not only was he a great surgeon, he also had a great bedside manner. He seemed to know intuitively exactly what I needed – be it a pat on the back or a kick in the butt.

He kept me walking and using the breath-strengthening device. He also started me on his famous 'dog food diet' (soft and mushy) as my new digestive system began its adjustment. On November 13th he gave me a good pathology report and the next day I passed the barium swallow test to go home. But Dr. Orringer wanted me to stay in the Ann Arbor area for a week until he was sure the sutures would hold - saying they would then have 'a lifetime guarantee'. So I moved in with local friends, who were empty nesters.

The following weekend, when members of my family came for the Ohio State football game, they drove me back to my hometown where I spent the next three and a half weeks with family. I continued the exercises which Dr. Orringer recommended and as I trudged in the snow up the high hill outside their house, I used to imagine myself as a concentration camp survivor on an end-of-war death march. I kept saying to myself, "I'm going to make it; I'm going to make it." And I did.

During my stay with my family, I struggled with my weight as well as my energy level. My weight dropped from 157.2 on November 17th to 148.8 on December 5th, the lowest it had been since I was a kid. Despite the great care of my family (they were excellent cooks), I had real trouble adjusting to the loss of 80% of my esophagus and the top part of the stomach. Still, on November 27th my oncologist gave me a good report in my first post-op visit. Eleven days later on December 8th my cousin drove me to Ann Arbor for my second post-op with Dr. Orringer. He removed the feeding tube; from now on I was totally dependent on my swallowing mechanism and he dismissed me to the care of my physicians in Cincinnati.

Inclement weather delayed my return to my own home. On December 15th another snowstorm hit. That evening, the two-and-a-half year old granddaughter of my cousin (the one who always drove me to Ann Arbor for my appointments with Dr. Orringer), was critically injured in an accident. We didn't know whether she'd survive or if she did, whether she'd be permanently impaired.

Fortunately, she eventually fully recovered. It helped put my own problems in perspective. Suddenly they didn't seem very significant. I was a 67-year-old man most of whose life had passed and who knew what was happening to him while she was just a child whose life was just starting. Needless to say, the family spent a mighty grim Christmas.

The next day on December 16th I returned home for the first time since I left for my surgery in Ann Arbor over a month ago. On the way, my cousins took me to see my internist for the initial visit since my cancer diagnosis. She found I was anemic and recommended I see a nutritionist, which I scheduled for January 9th. While I was glad to be home, I was discouraged, despite the good reports from my oncologist and Dr. Orringer. It was all I could do to accomplish simple tasks such as making meals and doing laundry, and there was much I wanted to do.

A considerable backlog had accumulated during my treatments. I had some 90 holiday cards to write, mainly to distant friends, and I wanted to include a personalized message on each of them, as I had in the past. Also, I had my mom's estate to settle. While I started on both, I accomplished little on either, seeing my attorney on December 29th but not completing the task until over a year later.

On January 9th I saw both my nutritionist and my oncologist. The nutritionist came first, and as I sat in her full waiting room, I noticed her overweight patients casting admiring glances at me as if I were some sort of 'success' story, while I thought I looked like death warmed over. She gave me some good recommendations, which I cleared with my oncologist, whom I saw next. I told him that I was discouraged with my progress; the difficulty in gaining weight and my low energy level. He assured me that I was doing fine. My blood tests were good, and I'd even gained a little weight. He emphasized that I had one of the most complicated surgeries possible, and it would take me three to six months before I started to feel like my old self again.

As I ate better, I felt better and gained weight, but my swallowing problems returned and, I feared, so had the cancer. On January 21st after a particularly traumatic time with food stuck in my reconstructed esophagus, I called Dr. Orringer's office. Being Saturday, it was closed, and I was referred to the Thoracic Surgery resident on duty. He told me the problem was common after esophagectomy and Dr. Orringer could easily correct it, doing it in his office without anesthetic. So on Monday I made an appointment and on January 26th I drove by myself to Ann Arbor.

To my amazement he did the dilation with only a numbing spray by inserting a few tubes of increasing size down my throat. He explained that scar tissue from the surgery was causing the problem, and the procedure might need to be done again later, raising the possibility of having me do it myself. This was something which was apparently unknown in Cincinnati, as was his dilation procedure.

Shortly after my return home, food again started to get stuck. So I called Dr. Orringer's office, but on learning that my gastroenterologist could do it using the tubes which Dr. Orringer recommended, I opted to have it done closer to home. On February 21st my gastroenterologist performed the second dilation but he did it after I was completely anesthetized (which happened on every one done in Cincinnati). When I awoke, he reported that I had scar tissue, and it would probably need to be done several more times, scheduling the next dilation for March 28th. Five days before that appointment I ended up in the emergency room and was hooked up with intravenous feeding to prevent dehydration. The following Monday a hospital gastroenterologist (I had to tell him not to use the balloon method, which he later said would have been easier) performed the procedure, again under a total anesthetic. On awakening, I was told that the esophagus was badly irritated but showed no signs of cancer and that I'd probably need to have the procedure done every three weeks for a year. A little over a week later on April 4th I needed it done again.

The day before the procedure on the 4th, I saw my oncologist. He urged me to contact Dr. Orringer about having future ones done in Ann Arbor. I was in the process of making the arrangements when I contracted a bad case of shingles. The physician assistant to my oncologist commented that I'd certainly had 'a lot of setbacks' on my road to recovery. So I had to have my 5th and 6th dilations on April 25th and May 25th done in Cincinnati, again, under a complete anesthetic. At my next appointment with my oncologist, he gave me a good report on my CT scan and noting my shingles had healed he urged me to contact Dr. Orringer, which I did.

On June 6th my cousin's wife (the nurse) and I traveled to Ann Arbor so I could be dilated for the seventh time this year (but only the second time by Dr. Orringer). This time he didn't even use the numbing anesthetic saying he learned from the first that my gag reflex was limited. After inserting the first two tubes, he let her do the third. She described it as easier than putting a feeding tube down a patient's nose into the stomach. He told us that if I had further difficulty we should return for instruction on how we could do it ourselves.

Two months later on August 17th, after I'd had some further difficulties, we drove back to Ann Arbor so Dr. Orringer could instruct us on using the French-Maloney dilator tube. After showing us how and letting us do it, he recommended we start by performing it every day for a week and then every other day, then every third day, etc. until the scar tissue became elasticized.

Within two weeks my nurse friend and relative taught me how to do the dilation myself so I no longer needed to stop at their home before breakfast. On one of my next visits to my oncologist I brought the French Maloney dilator tube with me, so he could show his staff, who had never seen one before.

My progress was easy afterwards. I ate better and gained weight, but never as much as before contracting cancer. I leveled off at 175 lbs.; 20 lbs. less than before it hit, which seemed ideal for my 5" 10½" frame. When my weight fell below 195 my blood pressure problem gradually disappeared until I no longer needed medication. The intervals between my self-dilations increased from days to weeks to months to years. My last was done approximately two years ago as a precaution in preparation for a foreign trip. The acid reflux attacks that plagued me early in my recovery gradually decreased in number and intensity, so they are no longer much of a problem.

Two years after my surgery the port for delivering chemo was removed, and the intervals between my oncology appointments grew from six weeks to three months to six months, to a year. Finally, on April 6, 2011, my oncologist dismissed me as a patient, saying he never wanted to see me again, which was a compliment.

In the 10 years since my cancer diagnosis, I have led an active life. I have traveled widely in the U.S., Europe, and Latin America. I have remained active in my community: church, local historical society, and city commission. I have also been able to be present at joyous occasions such as christenings, graduations, weddings, and high school and college reunions and at sad ones such as funerals which are an important part of life - my mother's side, being Irish, always has the best funerals because they are 'Celebrations of Life'. And I continue to visit Ann Arbor every fall to see friends and attend major U of M home football games. Life has been good. (I only wish our football team had been better.)

Ironically, cancer treatments have improved both my life expectancy and my quality of life. In many respects, I'm in better shape now than I was before. At my six-month check-up last week with my internist, I registered a weight of 175 lbs., blood pressure of 124/80, and pulse of 64 (at 77 plus years of age). I also take only one prescription medication for glaucoma. Things that once concerned me no longer do. Each new day is a blessing. Thinking I was going to die, I told my family and friends how glad I was that they were part of my life, and I learned who my real friends were. My dad used to say, "You won't know who your friends are until you need a friend". I also tied up the loose ends of my life. So, if I step off the curb tomorrow and get hit by a bus I will be at peace with the world. All of this would have been impossible without the support of family and friends and the excellent medical care I received, especially from Dr. Orringer.

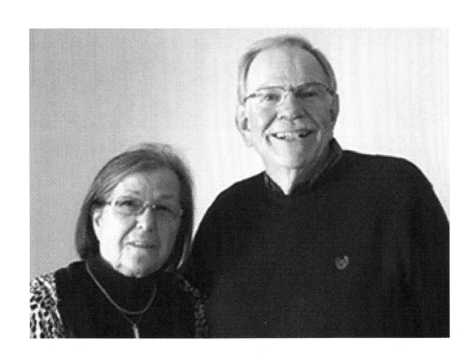

Carolyn and Paul E.

Chapter 8

My Esophagectomy Story

by Paul E.

My name is Paul E. I am a married man now 70 years old. In early 2005 I went to my primary care physician because I was having increasing difficulty swallowing. My primary care physician diagnosed me as having acid reflux and prescribed medication. When that did not help I went back to her in April and she sent me for a barium swallow esophagram test. That test showed that I had an almost complete blockage of the esophagus at the gastric junction, where the esophagus joins the stomach. She then scheduled me for an upper endoscopy exam in early May.

While I waited for that exam date I talked to a family member who had a friend who had a similar situation. This required her friend to have a periodic endoscopic procedure to stretch the opening to the stomach from the esophagus. While this was not something to look forward to, it certainly seemed manageable. I went to the endoscopic exam expecting that this is what I would hear.

When I awoke from the anesthesia after the endoscopic exam, the doctor who had performed the procedure came in and told my wife and me that I had cancer. This came as a complete shock. I had thought that I knew what was coming and never expected this news. We had to wait for the biopsy results to be sure, but when they came in I was diagnosed with Stage III esophageal adenocarcinoma cancer.

This was a very frightening diagnosis. When we researched this condition on the internet we were stunned by the information we found out about the low survival rate for this type of cancer. Up to this time, I had never even heard of esophageal cancer. I was immediately referred to an oncologist who would plan my treatment. He told me that I would require chemotherapy and radiation therapy followed by surgery to remove the affected area of my esophagus.

I was fortunate in that I had a lot of family support throughout this. My niece is a Naturopathic Doctor and she offered nutritional advice that helped me prepare for the chemotherapy and radiation therapy sessions that I would have to undergo. My brother and his wife are trained Reiki practitioners and they gave me Reiki healing treatments while I was receiving the chemotherapy treatments. This helped me deal with the stress. They also helped us research available treatments and identify treatment facilities I should consider.

I found it difficult to decide where to seek treatment under the weight of the terrifying diagnosis. At this time I also started a "Gratitude Book". This was a journal where every day I wrote down things that I was grateful for. This helped me realize that I had a lot of good things in my life along with the cancer.

Five sessions of chemotherapy treatments started immediately. My oncologist also referred me to a thoracic surgeon for removal of the tumor after the chemotherapy and radiation had shrunken or killed it. The first meeting with the surgeon was very discouraging because he told us that this would take my life. He told me that he would work with another surgeon, who would open my abdomen and prepare the stomach to be pulled up to the neck. I would spend about two weeks in intensive care after the surgery. I asked him how many of these operations he had performed and he told me that he had performed a few. I then asked him who was the best at this and performed the most of these surgeries. He told me that would be Dr. Mark Orringer at the University of Michigan and he offered to give me a referral to him for a second opinion.

Our research told us that the best surgical care for esophageal cancer was right in our backyard from Dr. Orringer at the University of Michigan. Dr. Orringer agreed to see me and we scheduled an appointment. At that meeting Dr. Orringer described in detail what he would do and told me that I would go to my room after the surgery instead of intensive care and that I would be up and walking the next day. I would probably be out of the hospital in seven or eight days. After that meeting we were more encouraged and decided that I would have Dr. Orringer perform my surgery.

At this point my wife and I decided that regardless of the insurance coverage and restrictions, I would go wherever I had to in order to get the best treatment. At this time the insurance plan I had would not cover me at the University of Michigan, but I was very fortunate in that because since I had been with my current insurance company for over a year, I was eligible to switch insurance companies. I switched to Blue Cross and Blue Shield effective the first of August and Dr. Orringer performed the surgery on August 15, 2005.

I was not aware of the Esophagectomy Support Group at the University of Michigan while I was going through all this, but family members put me in touch with two other people they knew personally who had survived esophageal cancer. They both had gone through treatment regimens similar to mine and had surgery to remove the esophagus and pull the stomach up. Both were doing well and happy with the quality of their lives. I was very encouraged by my contact with both of these people. Because I found it so helpful to talk to survivors during my treatment and before the surgery, I continue to participate regularly in the Esophagectomy Support Group at the University of Michigan.

After a few weeks of rest from the chemotherapy and radiation treatments Dr. Orringer performed a Transhiatal Esophagectomy (THE) plus Cervical Esophagogastric Anastomosis (CEGA) on me. As preparation before the operation I walked three miles per day as requested by Dr. Orringer to get my body in shape. This got to be quite difficult to do toward the end of the chemotherapy and radiation regimen. I also used a spirometer regularly to get my lungs in shape. This was also a request by Dr. Orringer.

This preparation paid off as I was able to get out of bed and walk the day after the surgery. The operation went very well and I do not recall having any significant pain. After the surgery, I was greatly relieved when Dr. Orringer told me that I did not have cancer; the pathology report showed that all the margins were clear, indicating that he removed the entire tumor. I went home from the hospital eight days after my surgery in the care of my wife, Carolyn, who deserves much of the credit for my good recovery.

I had a feeding tube when I left the hospital, but we never needed to use it as I was able to eat enough regular food to keep me going. It was not easy because I did not experience a feeling of hunger and most food had no taste at first, but that got better over time. Carolyn kept very close track of what I ate and kept encouraging me to eat so that I got enough calories.

I never had any trouble speaking or swallowing normally after the surgery. I was checked regularly by my oncologist every six months for five years after the surgery and there is no evidence of any recurrence or spread of the cancer.

I was retired at the time of my surgery, but I was able to resume all my normal activities and travel after about six weeks. During the whole process I lost about ninety pounds and most of it has stayed off. I can eat about anything I want - just not too much of it at any one time. I am pretty careful to eat mostly healthy foods. I also have to eat something fairly frequently, but that has not stopped my wife and I from traveling by automobile and airplane and staying in motels and eating all our meals in restaurants for extended periods. If I do manage to eat too much at a single sitting, my usual reaction is a feeling of fatigue, which usually passes within an hour or so. I can now lie down and sleep laying flat on a regular bed. My energy level has long since returned to normal and I am able to do about anything I want. I play golf regularly during the season. I pay pretty close attention to eating healthy now and I usually go for acupuncture once per week. I am very satisfied with my high quality of life since the surgery.

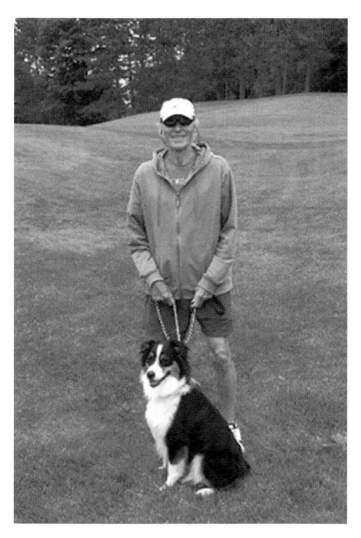

Peter H.

Chapter 9

My Toughest Marathon

by Peter H.

This is a story that I never imagined would be mine to tell. I have been a health conscious athlete and vegetarian since high school. I have spent most of my 68 years trying to do the best things I can to stay in shape because being active has always been so important to me. I started running in junior high, competed in high school (including setting school records in the mile and other distances), and I was an eight-time All American distance runner in college. I never stopped competing throughout my Navy service (I am a Vietnam-era vet). Throughout my adult life, I have run countless track and road races including forty marathons. No one could have been more surprised than I was to hear that I had cancer.

Like others I have spoken with, my diagnosis came after I complained about difficulty swallowing, particularly when eating bagels or bread. Drinking anything carbonated also really started to bother me. I waited to see my doctor and even delayed in talking about it with my wife, Robin, for almost a year. Once I mentioned my problem, she convinced me to see the doctor. At first it seemed I might have some kind of hiatal hernia or a stiffening esophagus but a swallow test and follow-up endoscopy in June of last year clearly gave the sobering news. I had a Stage III tumor in my lower esophagus and it was spreading into my stomach. On the one hand, I was shocked and on the other, by this point I was prepared for the worst.

I began a five-week treatment of chemotherapy and radiation in early August 2014. I continued to run and rode my bike to radiation treatment every day. While I was able to continue the cycling all the way until my last day of this treatment, about halfway through the doctors suggested I shift to walking rather than daily running as I was tiring myself out more than I was helping.

I do think that my general fitness level helped me get through the treatments with reduced side effects. At the same time it was clear to me quite early on that the chemo and radiation were having an effect on my tumor. Within a couple of weeks of starting this treatment, my swallowing improved and I could eat more easily than I had in some time. However, by the later stages of the treatment my esophagus was feeling the impact of the radiation and it became harder for me to swallow again.

Over time I realized that the anti-nausea drugs and painkillers that were offered were helpful to me and I needed to take advantage of them in spite of my life-long aversion to taking drugs. Before cancer I was not on any regular medications, which I have been told was unusual for someone my age. Throughout the treatment, the oncology and radiological oncology doctors and other health care providers were supportive and reassuring. They have difficult, demanding jobs but made me feel that they had time for my questions and concerns and that they cared about my outcome. I will be forever grateful for that.

The five weeks of chemo and radiation were extremely difficult, often because I only learned the hard way from experience what I needed to do to get through it. I alternated between constipation and diarrhea that I found difficult to keep in balance. That led me to be dehydrated so severely that I was hospitalized for a few days mid-treatment. My taste for food changed constantly and I would only be able to eat some things for a short period of time before they made me so nauseated that I could no longer eat them.

Throughout this process, one of my concerns was potential weight loss. At 6 feet tall I have weighed 150 pounds since high school, leaving me little room to spare for any loss. My first visit to the esophageal cancer support group in September was very helpful at answering questions but hearing how much weight most patients had lost during their treatment and post-surgery really concerned me. I knew I would have to work really hard to keep my weight up.

In the weeks after chemo and radiation leading up to my surgery, I started to feel better and was able to eat more normally. I was able to take a trip up to northern Wisconsin to our family place for some fishing and to relax before preparing for surgery.

My surgery took place on October 29, 2014. My surgeon, Dr. Carrott, had my full trust as a dedicated and skilled expert. He performed a nine-hour surgery successfully removing the lower portion of my esophagus and my entire stomach with only four laparoscopic incisions and a partial thoracotomy under my arm. I was hospitalized for eleven days following the operation. My wife stayed constantly by my side and slept in my room with me every night. We were very glad that we had made arrangements to board our dog for two weeks so that she had no other outside commitments. She also took a month off of work, which helped to reduce her stress and allowed her to focus on helping me recover. Many of my friends and family also offered amazing support to me.

I was out of bed and up walking the day after my surgery. I did have a few complications that were things we understood might happen from the patient education we received in advance. My intestines were slow to revive after the long surgery and use of narcotic painkillers immediately after the surgery. Therefore, I had to stay in the hospital a few extra days until I was able to eat properly. I started on a liquid and then "soft mushy" diet while in-patient. My initial post-op swallow test indicated that things looked good in terms of reconnection and after that I was sent home with a J tube for supplemental feeding. On my first day home I was able to walk to the corner coffee shop and back and thought I was on my way to a smooth recovery.

Within a few days, however, I noticed some difficulty swallowing again. I was experiencing restriction in my esophagus as other patients had described to me at the support group. An additional swallow test confirmed that there was some stricture and also some indication of a small leak. A stint was inserted to allow this to heal. I was required to stay on a liquid diet for the three additional weeks that the stint was in place and my weight continued to fall. Without solid food I also did not feel that I was gaining strength in spite of high caloric intake through the J tube.

Eventually I was re-hospitalized just before the Christmas holiday for an infection in my chest that was related to the stint and required a five-day in-patient stay on antibiotics. At the lowest point my weight dropped to near 130 pounds. Dr. Carrott, the physician assistants, and nurses on 4-C worked very hard to help me pull through this infection. Once this was cleared up I was able to eat a wider range of foods and my weight started to climb. I also felt much better on solid food and was able to increase my walking every day.

On January 9, 2015 my J tube was removed and I was cleared to begin jogging and doing some light exercise along with eating a regular diet. After that I started to feel the best I had felt since before my diagnosis. I am now an additional eight weeks out past that point. I no longer am seeing Dr. Carrott on a regular basis. My next visit to the oncologist is in April. I am doing the best I can to live in the present and not worry about what the future might mean for my health. My wife is retiring from her position at the University at the end of April and we plan to spend much of the summer in northern Wisconsin, if possible.

The care I received at the University of Michigan was exceptional. The staff was attentive and professional. Not only did my surgeon, Dr. Carrott make me feel personally cared for, but the other members of the team were also supportive. Dr. Orringer came to visit me in my hospital room every day to check on me and spent time at my bedside encouraging me. The nurses were so committed to my recovery and very understanding about how difficult and frustrating it is to be in such a vulnerable state.

I know that my life will never be exactly as it was before cancer. I will have to be very careful about my diet for the rest of my life. I sleep with my head elevated on a wedge pillow at night. I am working hard to regain the strength that I had before my illness. Because of the somewhat unusual complete removal of my stomach, I will require a monthly B-12 shot.

And I will remain thankful for every day that has been given to me by this miraculous medical procedure.

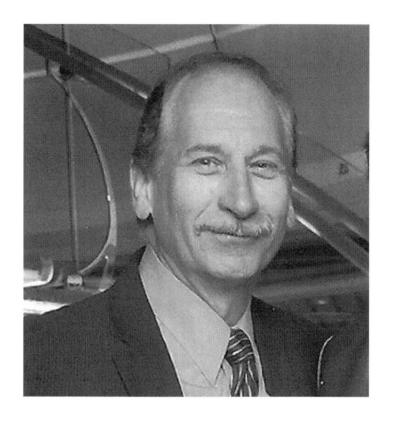

Russ P.

Chapter 10

Surviving Esophageal Cancer

by Russ P.

My name is (Russell) Russ P. I am married and have two sons. I am 55 years old. My story begins roughly 35 years ago. I can remember when I was in my 20's having mild heartburn. I would sometimes wake up choking or gasping for air. I tolerated this ailment for many years. For heartburn I just chewed antacids and this relieved it until the next time.

On a company golf trip in 1996, my hotel roommate, a co-worker, asked me the following morning if I realized that I was snoring really bad and at times was gasping for air. I did not realize this and went for a sleep study in 1997. I was diagnosed with obstructive sleep apnea. The CPAP machine, which I still use today, has prevented heart disease and other life threatening diseases.

Fast-forward twelve years to September, 2009. After so many years of ignoring GERD and heartburn, the effects this took on my esophagus were about to be discovered. I was on vacation and during lunch one day I was having a hard time swallowing my lunch. This was a strange feeling and during my colonoscopy consultation, I told the Gastroenterologist about my swallowing problem. He said that we should have an EGD scope performed.

During this exam the doctor found that seven percent of my esophagus was blocked by a mass. He did a biopsy. I received a call about a week later and found out that the mass was cancerous. The shock of that news was so devastating.

After the initial shock, I started to do research on the cancer. The initial consultation with the Henry Ford Hospital oncologist started the process. I started a journal and did more research. The recommended protocol for this type of cancer is chemotherapy, radiation and surgery. After a few weeks, the oncologist wanted me to talk with three surgeons. I made three consultation appointments with the surgeons. After consulting with the University of Michigan Radiation Oncology, Oncology, and Dr. Mark Orringer, I decided that I would have all three procedures done at U-M.

In November of 2009 I started my chemo and radiation treatments. The radiation was done two times per day for four weeks. Chemo was done for three weeks and I was not able to have the last chemo treatment because of a low white blood cell count. My chemo and radiation treatments were completed and during the CT scan it was determined that I had two small pulmonary embolisms. I never had any symptoms and was instructed to go to my primary care physician immediately to get blood thinners. This delayed my surgery as the doctors had to be sure I was healthy enough for the surgery.

The date was now set. I would have my surgery on March 10, 2010. I walked three miles a day and used my Spirometer to get my lungs prepared. Dr. Mark Orringer was my surgeon. During the surgery, Dr. Orringer had a hard time freeing up the tumor, but he persisted. The esophagus was removed and I spent the next seven days in the hospital. My recovery was very good. The pathology results showed all cancer was removed. What great news!

Today, I am a cancer survivor and am very grateful for the nurses, doctors, and the entire staff at the University of Michigan hospital. They truly saved my life. The many prayers from family and friends sure helped and for that I am grateful, as well.

My quality of life is very good and I am leading a normal life. I did lose about 40 pounds during treatments and surgery, but my weight has leveled off now and I am eating normally. This 'New Normal' means eating smaller meals more frequently.

Cancer can be beat! Think positive! I did!

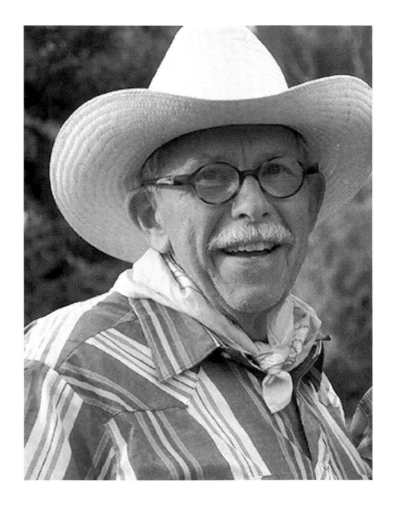

Stephen P.

Chapter 11

My Journey:
Esophageal Cancer To
Transhiatal Esophagectomy ("THE")

by Stephen P.

Looking back, it started with hiccups, simple hiccups. And some reflux. I mentioned these symptoms to my internist, and he was keen enough to suggest a scope and a biopsy. Another surgeon friend strongly encouraged me to complete the tests. Within about 48 hours of the procedures, they knew enough to suggest that I might have cancer. It would take a biopsy to confirm. Diagnosis: Esophageal cancer.

I live in Toledo and so far all of my medical care was done in the Northwest Ohio area. I consulted with local surgeons, and also discussed my plight with many friends. I am a pediatric dentist, so I called everyone in the medical profession that I knew. Every option, or so it seemed, was discussed: Chemo, radiation, and radical surgery.

The more people I talked to in Toledo and nationwide, a dominant theme emerged. Go and meet with Dr. Mark Orringer of the Thoracic Surgery department at the University of Michigan. I started to look into his research. I watched a video of the THE-CEGA procedure. It seemed cutting edge and based in research and practical successes. I also contacted a couple of patients who had the same surgery. I knew I had to consult with him.

And then came roadblock number one.

Because Dr. Orringer developed "THE-CEGA" procedure and his success was widely known, it was difficult to get an appointment with him. Dr. S., an ardent Ohio State fan and my internist, also agreed to write a letter of referral. Finally, I had an appointment with the team.

All the while, I was continuing with my treatment plan in Toledo, because all of the surgery prep would also be needed for Dr. Orringer if he decided to take on my case. I gathered all my records, had a barium swallow, a CT scan, and a PET scan. I needed a trans-esophageal ultrasound, and at this time it was only being performed at the University of Michigan, so we travelled up there to have it.

In late February of 2007, we went to the U-M Thoracic Surgery Clinic to meet Dr. Orringer. He had reviewed the pathology slides, lower GI film, and referral letters prior to our visit. Meeting with Dr. Orringer confirmed my decision that I wanted to work with him and have the CEGA procedure.

In March, I was scheduled for a chemotherapy consult and a radiation oncology consult. The cancer tumor board review usually happens every Friday afternoon. Following the Board review I was accepted as a patient of Dr. Orringer for 'THE CEGA.' I am so thankful. My diagnosis was Stage III adenocarcinoma of the lower end of the esophagus at the junction of the stomach. I was scheduled for surgery.

To get ready for the surgery I had to do breathing exercises, walk three miles per day, have chemo, radiation and get strong. This took the month of April. We live an hour and a half southeast of Ann Arbor, so we stayed at a hotel near the hospital during the week.

At the time of our first appointment with Dr. Orringer, Leah - one special clinic nurse - overheard Mary and I discussing how long I would be off work. Leah asked, "Why?" Mary replied, "Our youngest daughter is getting married in late July. Steve wants to dance at her wedding." I think at that time Leah knew we'd be at the wedding.

Chemo was tough! I remember the hand and foot massages during Chemo treatment. I remember I was told to visualize the radiation beams 'sinking into the cancer cells.' I used deep breathing exercises to help during treatment - thanks to Dr. W. The taste of food diminished. Eating was becoming more difficult. Liquid protein supplements were needed. Luckily, I had no major mouth sores. Getting used to the PICC line and chemo pump was do-able.

In May, three months after the diagnosis, chemo and radiation was over. Dr. Mark Orringer outlined our plan: Rest, get your labs improved, keep walking and breathing as instructed. Surgery will be the 1st week of June.

Finally, it was the big day. I slept during the surgery. I was in my hospital room that night. I remember the next morning with many tubes hanging from every part of my body. I felt like I was 'side-swiped by a semi.' Day one after surgery, I moved out of bed to sit in a chair for 10 minutes so the bed could be made. A couple of hours later someone came in and said, "I'll help you walk to the door." Wow, I was moving already!

That evening, with support, I walked to the nurse's station. My room was almost across the hall, but still, it was a step in the right direction (pun intended). The epidural helped to control my discomfort. Tubes were removed almost daily, except for my J-tube. On day three or four, I was able to walk to the Esophageal Support Group meeting down the hall. Since my surgery was in June, I even walked outside on the patio with 'my pole' to have lunch. I just kept walking and walking. I continue to walk a lot today.

Before I could be discharged, I needed a swallow study. On the morning of the swallow study wheel chair transportation was late. As the nurses were re-checking my heart rate, I was in atrial fibrillation. The physician assistants converted my rhythms. I did pass the swallow test but had to stay another day. Discharge and follow up was uneventful.

It goes without saying 'everyone is different', but having a positive attitude sure helped me! After my discharge, I continued to meet with the nutritionist and the support group because they offered valuable hints to smooth my transition at mealtime. In fact, eating small meals six or seven times per day became routine. I found that certain foods were 'triggers for dumping'. I avoided sweet foods such as maple syrup, brownies and beer. For me, spicy foods like pepper or wasabi woke up my the taste buds. I did lose about 60 pounds before surgery. Now, my weight has been constant at 162 to 168 for the last five years. I look for sources of protein, avoid most sweets and share entrees when Mary and I eat out. I eat everything, but in smaller portions.

I did dance the polka at my daughter's wedding in late July 2007. I was cancer free and dancing! Now, six years later, I am still dancing, blowing glass, traveling and practicing dentistry.

To this day, I know Dr. Orringer and his multi-talented team in Ann Arbor, Michigan is the best! I am also here today because of unselfish support from my wife, Mary, and our daughters and their husbands, as well as encouragement from my partner, Michael P. Glinka, DDS and our pediatric dental office staff during my four months of medical leave.

Our Esophageal Support Group is one of a kind!! It is low key, interactive, and has great staff leadership and physician support. It is available to those who have been, are, or will be in my (dancing) shoes.

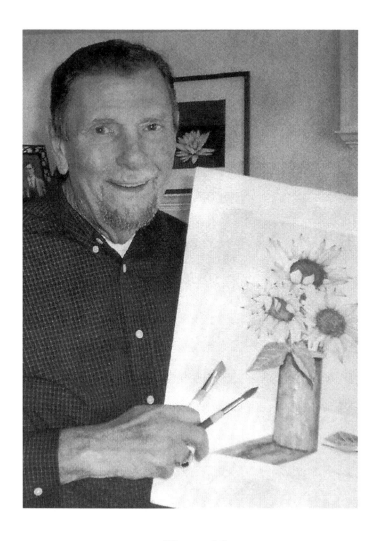

Vincent M.

Chapter 12

Esophagectomy Story

by Vincent M.

When asked to write my story by the Clinical Care Coordinator, Thoracic Surgery section of U-M Hospital, my first response was that I did not want to scare anyone. I then wondered why I haven't done it sooner and what do I want to convey to the readers.

First: If you experience acid reflux for whatever reason, have a check-up - an upper endoscopy - for GERD, Barrett's Esophagus, or tumors. If it is Barrett's Esophagus, get an annual biopsy to check for cancer. Don't assume you can just live with heartburn.

Second: If you have cancer in your esophagus and need an esophagectomy, ask everyone to pray to God to help you and your surgeons. I can tell you first hand that the Lord's will and the doctors' skill pulled me through many scary times. I'm here today writing this because of the dedication and skill of my surgeons and doctors and the enormous power of prayer to our Lord.

My cancer story begins with many years of acid reflux in my esophagus. I thought this was a common problem and for many years treated it with various antacids. Bad eating habits also did not help the problem. It was 2005 when I developed and had treated a bleeding ulcer in the lower portion of my esophagus. On inspection after the cauterization cleared up, I was told I had a condition called Barrett's Esophagus. This in itself did not mean I had cancer, but it could cause it. So, every year I had an upper endoscopy with biopsies taken. The years 2005, 2006, and 2007 showed no dysplasia, but in 2008 the biopsies showed early stage microscopic esophageal cancer.

My family doctor suggested a thoracic surgeon at a local hospital. She recommended a minimally invasive esophagectomy using the stomach made into a tube and put in place of the removed (cancerous) esophagus. I had just turned 73 years old and I underwent various tests by other doctors for their permission to have the operation. The operation was scheduled for October 30, 2008.

It was suggested that I call Dr. Mark Orringer at U-M Hospital for a second opinion. I called his office and was told that he was not available until well past the date of my scheduled operation.

The operation was performed at a local hospital and went well into the evening of the 30th and the next morning they wanted me to get out of bed and sit in a chair. I then collapsed and had emergency surgery performed because all of my organs were failing. The stomach being used for an esophagus became infected and the blood supply was compromised. The emergency surgery removed the stomach tube esophagus, a feeding tube was inserted into my small intestines, and a throat stoma was made with a bag to be changed two times a week. I stayed on the feeding system until well after I had a colon interposition at U-M. More about that operation later.

The emergency surgery saved my life. The surgeon told my family before going into surgery that while we had lost our oldest son to heart failure six months earlier, she would do everything possible for us to not lose another family member.

From October 30, 2008 to November 12, 2008, I was in the Intensive Care Unit. I stayed on a ventilator until November 9th. Upon removal of the ventilator, I sang with my new, hoarse, deep voice, "Here's To All The Girls I've Known," to my wife. On November 11th I found out that I had Stage III kidney damage. From November 12th to the 19th, I was in Progressive Care with pneumonia and a bowel infection. From November 19th to December 1st, 2008, I was sent to a rehabilitation facility for rehab and while there I became severely dehydrated and was sent back to the hospital to complete my rehabilitation. On December 29, 2008 I was sent HOME.

I was still on the feeding tube and wore a bag at my throat to catch saliva and anything else I put in my mouth, like popsicles. At home I was under the care of visiting nurses three times a week. On January 20, 2009 I was readmitted to the hospital because of a bacterial blood infection. On the 29th, I was released HOME with a PICC line for three antibiotics. I stopped taking the last one on March 16, 2009. No more infections as of March 23, 2009.

I stayed on the bag and pump feeding system for 14 months, for 16 hours each day, from October 31, 2008 to December 3, 2009. All medicines in pill form had to be crushed and put in the bag. My wife got up in the middle of the night to refill the feeding bag with liquid food. It had to be refilled every four hours. My wife deserves a nursing certificate for all she learned and did for my recovery.

I was able to move around and do some walking for eight hours each day. Three emergencies happened while on the feeding tube: 1) Clogged, 2) Clogged and bleeding, 3) Tube fell out while taking a shower. I picked it up off the floor, rinsed it off and shoved it back in. Went to Emergency to see if it was in the right place; it was. Mouthwash did not work, so I put V8 juice in a 3oz cup, added six drops of Tabasco sauce and sipped it. It worked in clearing up my mouth and restoring my taste. It gave new meaning to the term 'Hot Lips'.

Our surgeon referred us to surgeon Dr. Andrew C. Chang, Thoracic Surgery, at U-M for colon interposition surgery. A portion of my colon was removed and used for an esophagus, connected directly to my small intestines for digestion. Small portions of food (no more than two cups) must be chewed very fine. The food flows by gravity through my esophagus-colon. (My 'New Normal'.)

This allowed me to get off the feeding tube system and swallow real food. The main concern of this type of operation is the possibility of leakage at the connections. Dr. Chang assured me that he was good at sewing. Before the operation was scheduled, I had the usual tests for risks such as heart, etc. On July 1, 2009, the U-M cardiologist found some aorta leakage, however, it was not a risk for surgery. I was also asked to build up my respiration with a spirometer and my endurance by walking a mile a day.

Surgery was August 6, 2009. Dr. Chang performed a successful 12-hour long colon interposition surgery. While in ICU on August 9,

2009, I went into cardiac arrest (0 heart rate), fought for breath and went into septic shock. Dr. Chang asked my wife to call in our family. It was late at night and my youngest son had just returned to Cincinnati. She prayed to our Lord and 15 minutes later they were able to stabilize me. Another example of the surgeon's skill and God's will.

I developed two types of pneumonia on August 15, 2009. I was in terrible pain in my gut. They finally got an ultrasound tech to the room and then, at 4:00am, I was taken down for a CT scan. On August 16, 2009 I had surgery to repair leakage and to disconnect the small intestine to what was left of my regular colon. The surgeon developed an ileostomy bag from the end of my small intestine. I had the ileostomy bag for eight months until reversal on April 30, 2010. The surgical wound was left open until August 18, 2009 and required surgery to close it. I was taken off the ventilator on the 21st and moved out of ICU on the 23rd. I went to Acute Rehabilitation at U-M on September 14, 2009 and was released HOME on September 22, 2009 with visiting nurses.

From the end of September 2009 through the end of April 2010 there were two emergencies: One for coughing up blood and another for internal bleeding causing a huge hematoma from shoulder to below the buttocks. I required five units of blood.

On December 2, 2009, Dr. Chang put a stent into a narrow part of the esophagus-colon, which was scarred by scar tissue from inadequate blood supply.

The 1st of May 2010, I underwent a 6.5-hour ileostomy reversal. The small intestine was reconnected to what was left of the colon. May 7, 2010 – HOME.

On August 10, 2010, the stent put in the narrow part of the colon had moved down and Dr. Chang was able to remove it from the esophagus-colon without surgery. He put in another shorter and wider stint that later traveled to the center of my small intestine. He removed it with a four-hour surgery on October 5, 2010. He said, "No More Stents". In fact, I think he added, "No More

Operations". He promised that as long as he could, he would take care of me.

This story would not be complete without relating the excellent home care I received from my wife, visiting nurses, and physical/occupational therapists. The last therapist was a wonderful guy that related to my Italian heritage. The last day when he felt I was able to endure it, we made homemade linguine on the kitchen counter with wheat flour that he brought. I supplied the eggs. He also brought his clamp-on pasta roller and cutter hand-cranked unit. That night my wife and daughter had the pasta. I froze my portion to eat after I felt sure I could swallow it.

This wraps up the major points in my Esophagectomy Journey. I must tell you that through it all I went in and out of atrial fibrillation, had far too many EGD's, blood tests, swallow tests, etc., etc. I still have Dr. Chang performing a surgical EGD with dilation on me every six months at the Medical Procedure Unit of U-M. I have accumulated many other doctors who are looking after me such as an internist (family), endocrinology (thyroid), cardiology (heart valve), vascular (atrial fib), and nephrology (kidneys).

I cannot lay flat on my back. If I do, the fluids from my mouth will not drain into my esophagus-colon, which passes food and fluids by gravity. I do not lie down until three hours after eating. I sleep on my back with my head and shoulders elevated on a wedge pillow. I've learned by trial and error what foods my small intestine can tolerate. If I eat the wrong food, such as lettuce, I will get painful cramps for three hours. When I eat more than two cups of food or have too much liquid with my meal, I'll experience what is called, 'the dumping syndrome'. I'd better find a restroom close by.

I'm somewhat restricted with travel plans for various reasons. All this is just part of my 'New Normal'. I will turn 80 years old this year and I'm thankful every day that I have the benefit of the Lord's will and the doctors' skills. Please pray for everyone having an esophagectomy.

I have learned to live with my 'New Normal'. It has been over six years since I had my esophagectomy, removal of my stomach, and a colon interposition. The learning experience has been mostly trial and error, but I always keep a happy, positive attitude.

If I disagree with someone, I like to ask them if they want me to swallow that? I don't have the stomach for it. I'll just go with my gut feeling and let it pass.

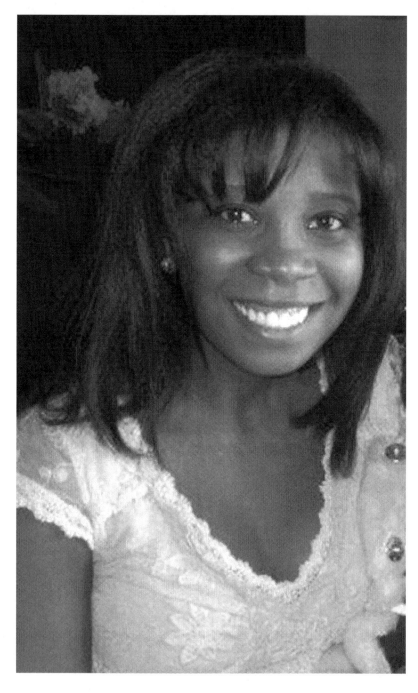

Tiffany Staal, BSN, R

Chapter 13

My Experience With the
Esophagectomy Support Group

by Tiffany Staal, BSN, RN

My name is Tiffany Staal and I am one of clinical coordinators working in the Thoracic Surgery clinic at the University of Michigan Health System. I was asked to write a short piece on my experience working with the Esophagectomy Support Group. To discuss the Support Group I feel I should start with my first experience with the thoracic surgery patient population. This is a story I share often with the support group members when we reflect on the standard of excellence Dr. Orringer has set here.

The year was 2008 and I was a travel nurse working on 4-C. I had been there a few months and had deemed myself worthy enough to take care of a transhiatal esophagectomy patient. I had never cared for an esophagectomy patient so I, of course, looked up the operation and was truly blown away. As I continued to read I realized that the Dr. Orringer I was reading about was *this* Dr. Orringer.

So, after a couple of hours I felt confident enough to go into the room and start my morning assessment on this particular patient and in walks Dr. Orringer. After he rounded on the patient, he asked me to step out of the room and asked if I understood everything that was done to the patient. I said, "Yes," (nervously, praying there wouldn't be a pop quiz). He said, "Good," and then proceeded to pick up a marker and draw the operation on the board for me. That was better than any website I could look up. After this I felt more confident and more excited about this unique patient population.

Fast-forward five years to 2013 when I began working in the Thoracic Surgery clinic. At this point I had taken care of my fair share of transhiatal esophagectomy patients. I was asked to cover the support group for the best predecessor a nurse could ask for, Lori Flint. She introduced me to the support group before she made her departure and although it was a mutual decision, I did not think I could ever be ready to fill her shoes.

My first group alone went well. I was anxious and nervous, hoping I wouldn't say something inaccurate and hoping (again) there wouldn't be a pop quiz. The group was as welcoming to me and all new patients as I could hope for. They have so much to offer to those newly diagnosed, scared people. I've learned a wealth of knowledge about the 'New Normal' and I apply it to my job daily. The members of the support group are exceptional, strong and great people. I am so glad I have been able to help keep the group going.

Sincerely,

Tiffany Staal, BSN, RN

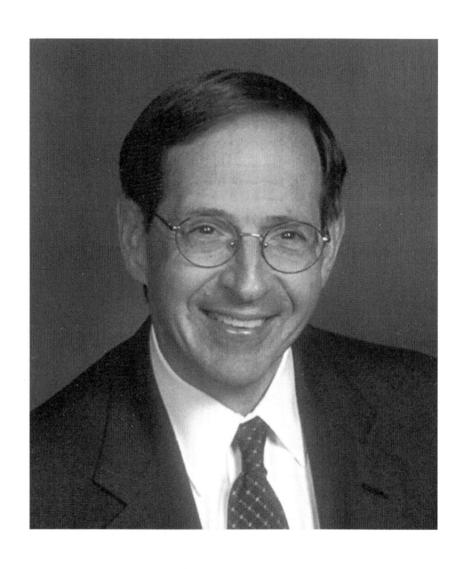

Mark B. Orringer, MD

Biography of Mark B. Orringer, M.D.

Mark B. Orringer, MD, attained both his bachelor's and medical degrees at the University of Pittsburgh, after which he completed residencies in general and thoracic surgery at The Johns Hopkins University in 1973. During his residency, he developed his interest in the surgical treatment of esophageal cancer as a senior registrar for the world-renowned thoracic surgeon, Mr. Ronald Belsey, at the Frenchay Hospital in Bristol, England.

Dr. Orringer was recruited by then Section Head, Professor Herbert Sloan, as assistant professor of thoracic surgery in 1973. By 1980, Dr. Orringer was promoted to Professor of Surgery. Reflecting his exemplary patient care and talent as an educator, Dr. Orringer was appointed as Section Head of Thoracic Surgery, remaining in this position until 2011.

Dr. Orringer challenged the paradigm for the treatment of esophageal cancer, for which patients had long-term survival of 15%. He rediscovered and refined the technique for transhiatal esophagectomy with cervical esophagogastric anastomosis, without thoracotomy (opening the chest), with the aim of reducing the complications and mortality associated with standard surgical approaches for esophagectomy, which required thoracotomy. Dr. Orringer also recruited Dr. David Beer to study the biology of thoracic malignancies, particularly both lung and esophageal cancer, and together they have built a research team that is internationally renowned for its contributions to esophageal and lung cancer biology.

Dr. Orringer has authored or co-authored over 250 peer-reviewed journal articles and 110 book chapters, edited five books and served on the editorial boards for several journals. He has served as president of both the Thoracic Surgery Directors Association and the Society of Thoracic Surgeons, as well as director of the American Board of Thoracic Surgery.

In addition to his distinguished academic and medical career, Dr. Orringer is known for his deep compassion and commitment to patient care and education. In 2014, the University of Michigan bestowed upon Dr. Orringer its highest professional title, the Cameron Haight Distinguished University Professor, in recognition of his academic contributions to the University and the nation. He has and continues to mentor generations of students, young surgeons and faculty.

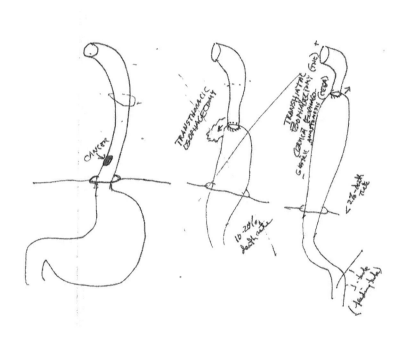

Drawing by Mark Orringer, M.D.

The Transhiatal Esophagectomy Procedure
("THE")

RESOURCES

For more information about esophageal cancer and resources for patients and caregivers, please see the websites below.

National Cancer Institute, at the National Institutes of Health
http://www.cancer.gov

Department of Surgery,
Thoracic Surgery at the University of Michigan:
"Esophageal Cancer – What is an Esophagectomy?"
http://surgery.med.umich.edu/thoracic/patient/what_we_do/esoph agus_cancer.shtml
(Short version of link: http://tinyurl.com/nay7elt)

Department of Surgery,
Thoracic Surgery at the University of Michigan:
"Transhiatal Esophagectomy (THE) – What is it?
Understanding Terminology"
http://surgery.med.umich.edu/thoracic/patient/what_we_do/esoph agectomy_faq.shtml
(Short version of link: http://tinyurl.com/oaarany)

Esophagectomy Support Group,
Thoracic Surgery at the University of Michigan
http://surgery.med.umich.edu/thoracic/patient/support_group.sht ml
(Short version of link: http://tinyurl.com/pc6546f)

CarePages
https://www.carepages.com

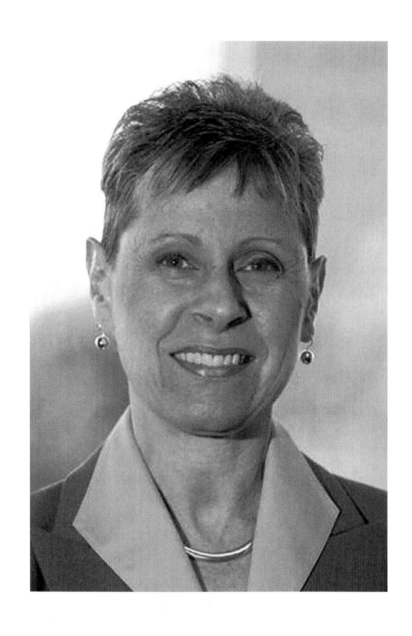

Ellen R. Abramson

ABOUT THE EDITOR

Ellen Abramson has been employed at the University of Michigan Health System for eleven years. She works as a development officer, raising funds to support medical research and education. Ellen has helped raise funds for several areas at the Health System, including Thoracic Surgery, Transplant Surgery, Orthopaedic Surgery, and Physical Medicine & Rehabilitation. In her role, she has the opportunity to help grateful patients and families, as well as alumni, make philanthropic gifts that have great meaning to them and make a meaningful difference in the world.

She holds a Master of Social Work degree from University of Michigan, and previous to her career in development, Ellen worked as a hospice social worker. She is deeply grateful for her many blessings, chief among them her remarkable husband and her wonderful daughters, son-in-law and grandchildren.

If you are interested in knowing how you can help advance research on esophageal cancer and other thoracic cancers and conditions, please contact the University of Michigan Health System Office of Medical Development at (734) 998-7705.

25715073R00061

Made in the USA
Middletown, DE
08 November 2015